the RAW50

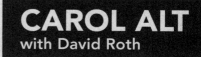

CAROL ALT
with David Roth

the
RAW 50

10 AMAZING BREAKFASTS, LUNCHES, DINNERS, SNACKS, AND DRINKS FOR YOUR RAW FOOD LIFESTYLE

CLARKSON POTTER/PUBLISHERS
NEW YORK

Library of Congress Cataloging-in-Publication Data

Alt, Carol,
The raw 50: 10 amazing breakfasts, lunches, dinners,
snacks, and drinks for your raw food lifestyle / Carol Alt
with David Roth.—1st ed.
Includes index.
1. Raw food diet—Recipes. I. Roth, David. II. Title.
III. Title: Raw fifty.
RM237.5.A467 2007
641.5'63—dc22   2006039185

ISBN 978-0-307-35174-6

Printed in the United States of America

Design by Laura Palese

10 9 8 7 6 5 4 3 2 1

First Edition

CONTENTS

FOREWORD BY NICHOLAS J. GONZALES, M.D.

When Carol Alt's first book, *Eating in the Raw,* proved to be so well received, I couldn't have been more pleased. I've been acquainted with Carol now for many years, and know how important it is to her to spread the word about good nutrition in general, and raw food in particular. *Eating in the Raw* did change lives, sometimes in very small ways, sometimes more profoundly. Since the book first came out, Carol has heard from many readers who reported that their health had been changed for the better by following some of the simple rules she outlined. Many wrote with gratitude that their energy had improved, their headaches had disappeared, the pounds had fallen away, the aches and pains had lessened, just by giving up the junk—the white flour, white bread, white sugar, the chemicals and the synthetics passed off as food—and instead turning to whole foods, clean foods, organic foods, and largely raw foods, with all the vital vitamins, minerals, and enzymes intact and untouched.

As she did with *Eating in the Raw,* Carol asked me if I would be willing to write the foreword to this new book. I was honored to do so. She and I continue to be eager to address the question we're commonly asked by those new to the raw food lifestyle: "Must I become a vegetarian to reap the benefits of this diet?" The short answer is no; while some who go raw do ultimately forgo animal products, including dairy, it is an individual choice based on what combination of foods makes one feel best.

I am also asked why raw food is beneficial to our health. The first time I talked at some length about enzymes, those intricate protein catalysts that allow the complicated reactions of life to occur efficiently and rapidly. I also pointed out that food not only provides proteins, fats, carbs, along with the health-promoting vitamins, minerals, and trace elements, but actually represents an excellent, though usually unappreciated, source of enzymes. In general, we don't think of food as a source of enzymes, though in fact, all food—whether animal or plant in origin—can provide large quantities of these life-supporting proteins. We can absorb these food enzymes for use as replacements for our own damaged and aging cellular catalysts. But here's the catch: Food can provide these beneficial enzymes only if it's raw.

In our office, my colleague Dr. Linda Isaacs and I don't recommend a single perfect diet that works for all. On the contrary, we prescribe a variety of diets for our patients, depending on individual metabolic needs. These can range from near vegetarian to largely red meat, with all variations in between. Such an approach, we realize, might be considered unusual, since in the nutritional world today, whether alternative or more conventional, dietary experts usually proclaim the value of one ideal diet. Too often, though, the perfect diet of one expert differs considerably from the perfect diet extolled by another, and the wars between the camps can become quite intense.

Many nutritional researchers maintain that all humans should eat vegetarian, or as close to vegetarian as possible. Such an approach reached full flower during the 1980s and 1990s, with the widely publicized dictates and popular books of vegetarian evangelists such as the late Nathan Pritikin, Dr. Dean Ornish, and those that promote the macrobiotic school of thought. All of these movements, though differing in the nuts-and-bolts specifics, subscribe to the belief that the less fat and the fewer animal products the better. For these thinkers and scientists, carbs are our true friend, the more the better, and animal fat and protein are the most insidious enemies, the "obvious root cause" of the epidemic obesity, diabetes, and heart disease afflicting most Western nations. Raw foods proponents such as the late Ann Wigmore, who for years ran a raw foods clinic in Boston, invariably tend toward the purely vegetarian: to these folks, raw means raw vegetarian, period.

On the other hand, there have been those, like the late Bob Atkins, as well as more conventional researchers such as Dr. Gerald Reaven from Stanford, who take the complete opposite tack. These physicians have warned and continue to warn that a high-carbohydrate, plant-based diet, particularly one heavy on refined sugar, refined white flour grains, synthetic trans-fats, and synthetic chemicals, is the true culprit behind obesity, diabetes, and heart disease—the very same problems the vegetarians blame on fat. Small wonder the consumer looking for simple guides for better health can experience nothing but confusion.

I have long thought that much of the angry dietary discourse might be resolved if only nutritional researchers would consider for a moment where our various ancestors came from, and the type of food they would have eaten. Historically, our antecedents occupied a variety of ecological niches, each providing a different type of food, from the Arctic Circle to the Equatorial jungles of South America. The foods available in each of these places vary considerably, and for humans to have existed in these locales, they would of necessity have had to survive on very disparate diets.

In the Arctic regions of Canada, Alaska, Siberia, and Greenland, winter lasts much of the year. Such a clime allows for no real summer of any consequence, and certainly not the significant growing season needed to nurture and harvest the plant foods most familiar to us: fruits, vegetables, nuts, seeds, and grains. In the Arctic, other than a few varieties of berries, plant foods suitable for human consumption simply do not exist. The Arctic does, however, provide an abundant supply of fatty animals, like caribou and bear, fatty fish, and for those near the sea, ocean animals such as seal and whale.

At the turn of the last century, the explorer and anthropologist Vilhjalmur Stefansson spent ten years studying the Inuit (previously known as Eskimos), living among them as one of the community, at a time in history when these famed hunters still lived their traditional and very isolated life. He summed up his observations and experiences in a series of very popular books published during the first half of the 1900s.

During his stay in the Arctic, he was astonished to find that the Inuit he observed lived on an all-meat diet consisting of about 80 percent fat—a way of eating that experts even in Stefansson's day claimed could not support human life. But eat meat the Inuit did, to their apparent great benefit. As Stefansson reported in his book *Not by Bread Alone* published in 1946, the Inuit he studied enjoyed extraordinary health, with apparent immunity to the diseases of civilization such as obesity, diabetes, heart disease, even arthritis and cancer. So impressed was Stefansson by the absence of cancer even among the most elderly Inuit that he wrote a book, first published in 1960, entitled *Cancer—Disease of Civilization*. Stefansson also noted that though the Inuit did cook some food, most of it was eaten raw or fermented. As a favorite treat, which Stefansson himself came to enjoy, his Inuit friends would bury fish or meat for weeks, let it sit, then come back and feast on the festering goo. Such natural processing, as strange as it may seem to us today, actually serves to improve a food's nutritional—and enzyme—content. In this way, the Inuit created their own unique superfood.

Dr. Weston Price, another pioneering researcher still underappreciated outside of the alternative world, was a dentist by training who spent seven years of his life during the 1930s traveling to remote regions of the world. During his extensive journey, Dr. Price studied diets of indigenous isolated peoples still living a traditional way of life and still eating a nonindustrialized diet. Over the years, he roamed from the Arctic home of the Inuit visited by Stefansson decades earlier to the depths of Africa, from the outer islands of Scotland to the high Peruvian Andes. In each place, he carefully observed not only the indigenous diet, but also the general health of the people, both those still following traditional nutritional practices, as well as those of the same background who had already begun to adopt the foods of "advanced" Western civilization.

Dr. Price put his findings together in a comprehensive book, *Nutrition and Physical Degeneration,* first published in 1946 and still available today. His findings suggested that humans in traditional settings eating traditional foods thrived on diets dictated by the available food, and not by one inviolate nutritional law. These diets ranged from the all-meat Inuit diet at one extreme to those of peoples living in milder climes that consisted of considerable amounts of plant foods, such as fruits, vegetables, nuts, seeds, and grains.

Furthermore, the people he observed used at least some form of animal food, be it meat, fish, eggs, or dairy—as in the case of the Masai, who drank up to a gallon of milk a day, or the high-mountain Swiss, who relied on cheese. That finding alone should long ago have put the "vegetarian is always best" argument to rest.

Price noted that the groups following their time-honored diets relied on food in its most natural form possible, processed minimally if at all. All of the food was grown locally, or in the case of animal products, obtained locally. This isn't an inconsequential observation: the storage and shipping of food invariably leads to loss of at least some nutritional value as well as flavor.

Interestingly, each of the groups Price studied had folk wisdom gleaned from their experience about the value of uncooked food, that raw foods provided nourishment more profoundly life sustaining than cooked versions of the same food.

In his travels, Price, a meticulous observer and a very sophisticated scientist, carefully documented the health histories of literally thousands of people and interviewed any Western physicians who might be living amongst these traditional peoples he studied. What he found, after years of hard labor, should have changed the course of modern dietetics and modern medicine. The common and chronic "diseases of civilization" that were already reaching epidemic proportions in Price's day—diabetes, heart disease, cancer, tuberculosis (at that time a deadly and common disease in the industrialized countries), and arthritis—seemed largely if not entirely absent among the populations he visited. Even those groups with what we might consider extreme eating practices (such as the Inuit, living on nothing but meat and mostly fat, or the Masai, surviving on raw milk and cattle blood) seemed to be in extraordinary physical shape.

As the years have passed, such studies have become nearly impossible to pursue, and Price's odyssey would not be feasible today. Even in the high Andes, Western foods have made insidious inroads, and few people anywhere follow what Price would have considered a "traditional" way of living and eating. But the points are valid, nonetheless:

- Humans have survived and thrived on very different diets, determined by locale and the available food source.

- No human group has lived traditionally on a vegetarian diet.

- Whole foods, whatever the specific diet, are always best.

- Local is better than that shipped from distant places.

- Raw is usually better than cooked.

Good nutrition can make a difference for everyone, in all of our lives. Good health can be our birthright and a way of life; good, optimal nutrition can potentially free us from many if not most of the diseases we most fear.

Hopefully, my foray into dietary history also reinforces the philosophy I advocate in our practice, that each of us may require a diet, depending on our genetic, nutritional, and cultural ancestry, that differs in important ways from that required by our neighbor, our doctor, or even our spouse. In terms of food, one size does not fit all.

But all of our many diets do include raw foods, to varying degrees. We rarely insist on all raw eating and in certain specific cases, we do allow considerable cooked food. First of all, we do see many patients with serious, often life-threatening diseases, and for some of these people, at least initially, we may recommend a fair amount of cooked food. Though heating destroys some vitamins, makes certain minerals like calcium less available, and destroys all enzymes, it does have the effect of breaking down cell walls in food, both plant and animal—in a sense predigesting the food. Some of our most debilitated patients tolerate cooked food more easily and make up for the nutrient and enzyme losses with additional supplements. Even in these cases, as the patient improves and as digestion normalizes, we gradually increase the percentage of raw.

In every case, though, we always insist the patients consume some raw foods. One easy, convenient, and very effective way to include raw food is through juicing, which virtually any patient can tolerate. A juicer will extract a plant's—be it fruit or vegetable—water and its various nutrients, which then separate out from the indigestible fiber. In the process, the vitamins, minerals, trace elements—and the vital living enzymes—are concentrated in the raw liquid. Freshly made juice provides nutrients and enzymes in a very dense, pure, and completely raw form—and with the fiber gone, the remaining juice is easily assimilated in the digestive tract, requiring very little effort or energy on our part. And though technically juice is not, in the purest sense of the word, a "whole food," since much if not most of the fiber is removed, it still provides a unique benefit, though the amounts need to be individualized. For our vegetarian patients, whose diets already provide large amounts of fiber, we often recommend four to six 8-ounce glasses a day, largely carrot-based. These patients tend to thrive on juice, often reporting a great boost in energy when they drink it. On the other hand, our carnivores do less well with juice, though for these folk we usually still advise a glass or two a day, but made only from root vegetables.

In addition to the diets we prescribe, we recommend a large number of supplements for our patients as part of our therapy. And all our patients, whatever their underlying problem, take an enzyme supplement specifically designed to replace those normally found in raw food. Though our supplement programs are largely enzyme based, in our protocols we prescribe for each patient specific combinations of vitamins, minerals, and trace elements, which, along with the enzymes, help regulate the thousands of reactions occurring in all our cells, tissues, and organs. We individualize each of these nutrient protocols as we do the diets, to address each patient's specific needs and health problems.

While prescribing a regimen of whole, mostly raw foods is just part of the overall treatment plan we prescribe our patients, we consider it a vital one, one without which the complementary supplements and diet modifications would fail to achieve their greatest benefit. Adhering to such food plans does take some adjustment for many of our patients, as it represents a significant change from the processed food, additive, refined sugar, and flour-based diets they are accustomed to. But the evidence in support of eating raw, whole, local, and unprocessed, some of which I've cited above, is persuasive.

Most of our patients are very unusual people. Though more orthodox researchers and physicians tend to view those who seek out "alternative" therapies and practitioners as rather dim-witted souls, easily manipulated by conniving, money-hungry victimizers, in fact, when scientists (such as Dr. Eisenberg from Harvard) have actually looked at such people, they turn out to be far more educated and intelligent than the average population of patients. We certainly find this to be the case in our own practice. Our patients overall think independently, look outside the box, and are often willing to take charge of their lives and their situation and make significant changes in order to improve their health. Though of course we are not always successful—no one could be, particularly with the population of patients who seek us out—we frequently do succeed, patients frequently get well and go on to enjoy productive, happy lives. Our successes give us the energy to keep going.

The following case study illustrates quite compellingly the impact of an enzyme-based diet on a patient suffering from metastatic breast cancer.

She had been in good health when a biopsy of a lesion in the left breast found on routine mammography confirmed cancer. Although her surgeon suggested a modified radical mastectomy, she insisted on a lumpectomy; the pathology report confirmed carcinoma. Radiographic studies showed no evidence of metastatic disease and consequently, since the disease seemed localized, her doctors suggested no further treatment.

She did well until her physician detected a mass in the opposite breast three years later. She underwent a lumpectomy shortly thereafter, and the tumor proved to be again cancerous, but this time more aggressive, having invaded the lymph nodes. Her doctors ordered an abdominal ultrasound, which revealed a mass in the right lobe of the liver. A needle biopsy confirmed the carcinoma had spread from the breast.

Metastatic breast cancer, particularly when it has invaded a major organ like the liver, is considered incurable. Chemotherapy and hormonal blockade can help some patients for a time, but invariably, even when the patient responds to treatment, the disease ultimately proves fatal.

The patient did agree to an aggressive multi-drug chemotherapy regimen, which she tolerated poorly. After completing three cycles of a projected six, she refused to continue because the side effects were so devastating, and her doctors had told her that even under the best of circumstances the therapy would not be curative. For several months, she did no treatment of any kind.

Word of mouth eventually led her to my office. She was quite ill at the time, suffering chronic pain in her liver, and initially she had a difficult course on her nutritional protocol. At times, the liver pain was so severe, she required morphine for comfort. She suffered episodes of fatigue and malaise for many months, before she finally began improving. When I saw her for a return evaluation a year after beginning treatment with me she was feeling much stronger and her abdominal pains had diminished greatly.

Unfortunately, she began to feel so well that she subsequently discontinued her protocol, assuming she was "cured." After suffering a recurrence of symptoms and the diagnosis of two masses in the brain consistent with metastatic cancer in 1991, she resumed her full nutritional program with renewed dedication. She quickly improved, and in April 1992, CT scans of both the head and abdomen revealed that the liver and brain tumors were gone.

Her story tells much about cancer, its course, and its control. We tend to think of this frightening illness in "all or none" terms; that is, if you don't exterminate every last malignant cell, the disease will spread aggressively and ultimately kill. But in our office, we have a different way of thinking about cancer, a disease we view as a potentially chronic problem that can be well controlled for years and decades, even if every last cancer cell isn't blasted out of existence. I usually tell our patients that managing cancer is like managing diabetes; a diabetic can live for a hundred years as long as he or she follows the prescribed diet and takes insulin. Invariably there will be ups and downs, medication doses will need to be changed, and if compliance falls off, certainly trouble follows quickly. Despite such pitfalls, many diabetics can lead fairly normal, productive lives as long as they stick to their treatment regimen.

This patient's diet protocol emphasizes plant foods in largely unlimited amounts: all the fresh fruits and vegetables she could eat, specified amounts of fruit and vegetable juices, raw nuts (particularly almonds, which have a mild anti-cancer effect), raw seeds and whole grains of various types and various forms. The diet also allows some limited animal protein, specifically eggs daily—which provide ideal protein, essential fatty acids, many vitamins and trace elements, and which do not, contrary to popular belief, raise cholesterol; whole-milk yogurt, which provides a rich supply of enzymes, easily digested protein, and many other nutrients; and fish, preferably a leaner variety such as sole, twice a week. However, poultry and red meat are strictly forbidden.

The diet requires that at least 70 percent of all food be consumed raw or very lightly cooked. Even in the case of cooked foods, such as breads, we recommend primarily the organic sprouted versions, such as those under the Ezekiel or Shiloh Farms label. Not only does sprouting increase the enzyme and overall nutritional content of a grain, but these particular breads are cooked at very low temperatures, to preserve most of the essential nutritional value.

It should be noted that, like all our cancer patients, this patient consumed in the range of 180 capsules a day, including large doses of pancreatic enzymes taken every four hours away from meals, as the main anti-cancer effect of the program. With different patients, and different diseases, we prescribe differing protocols, and this story is not intended to advocate a particular cure-all regimen for combating all diseases, or even all cancers. Rather I hope to make the point that good nutrition, specifically enzyme-based good nutrition, is a powerful tool, not just for those of us hoping to increase our energy or lose weight, but also for those diagnosed with serious illness. And, as much as we already know, thanks to scientists such as Weston Price, I believe that we're only at the beginning in terms of our understanding of what proper diet and whole foods living can do for all of us.

However, for those looking for help now in their own whole foods, raw foods journey, Carol's new book is a great place to start. Tested in the front lines of the kitchen, her recipes stick true to her nutritional message and provide a varied and tasty set of meals that will convince just about anyone that whole raw foods are indeed best.

NICHOLAS J. GONZALEZ, M.D. *(Cornell University Medical College), began his medical research career working under Dr. Robert A. Good, often called the father of modern immunology. Dr. Gonzalez currently practices in New York City, where he offers intensive nutritional therapies for patients with serious degenerative diseases such as cancer. The National Institutes of Health as well as Nestlé and Procter & Gamble have supported his research.*

INTRODUCTION

When I wrote *Eating in the Raw* my motivation was simple: I couldn't keep a secret. I had been eating nearly 100 percent raw for almost a decade. Raw food had literally changed my life, and permanently so, and I wanted to share what I had learned with everyone.

I have always loved to dispel people's long-held notions and to shatter their misconceptions. I've found that most people will attack what they don't know. Instead of doing their own homework, they'll follow like sheep whatever passing fad diet the media happens to pick up on. Remember the no-fat Pritikin diet and the no-carbs Atkins diet? What will happen when the fad becomes a no-protein diet? What will be left to eat?

As a former sheep, myself, I tried all those diets. I never lost weight, or if I did, I never could keep it off. Some of the diets actually made me sick. (I'll never forget throwing up frozen blueberries one winter when I was on a popular all-fruit diet!) When none of the trendy diets worked, I was left to my own devices. And I must say that on my own I didn't fare much better. While starving myself to try to lose weight, I'd gain weight if I ate a single potato! And along the way I gave myself hypoglycemia, too.

I had finally given up all hope, my ego's defenses were down, and I was at my wits' end. Then one day, God gave me—by way of two brilliant doctors, first Timothy Brantley and later Nick Gonzalez—what has become the key to my life, looks, and the longevity of my career.

What I found is that with just a few adjustments to what I was eating, mostly in the way that my foods were prepared, I could eat almost anything I wanted. And boy, did the food taste good—unbelievably good! My weight stayed perfect and I felt amazing too! Not only that; it cured the things that were literally ailing me. I still marvel.

Eating what other diet, living what other lifestyle, can you shamelessly have such a wide range of delicious foods and treats? None. It's only possible by eating the kinds of foods you find here in *The Raw 50*—by eating raw!

This was not a fad diet. Unlike many doctors and authors who create diets but don't practice them, or who promote diets but still look and feel horrible, once I started eating raw, I felt and looked great. At forty, I felt better than I had at twenty. People regularly came up to me and remarked that I looked better than I did in the 1980s, when *Playboy* magazine called me "the Most Beautiful Woman in the World." The title was something that always made me a little uncomfortable and may have been a bit of an exaggeration, but since I was feeling bad, it was a real shot in the arm.

Then I wrote *Eating in the Raw*. The subtitle of that book was "A beginner's guide to getting slimmer, feeling healthier, and looking younger the raw-food way." Based on the mail I received and the people who stopped me on the street to talk about how *Eating in the Raw* had changed their lives, the book accomplished what I had set out to do. It introduced people to the benefits of eating raw and showed them how to put raw principles into practice. It dispelled the common misconception that eating raw food means gnawing on a carrot and a stalk of celery and going hungry. The photo on that book's cover shows me standing beside an array of gourmet entrées and desserts. I'm holding a sundae that, I confess, I couldn't resist eating the moment after the photo was shot.

Since taking up the raw food lifestyle, I have never gone hungry and I have never seen my weight fluctuate, as I did when I was dieting while eating cooked food and constantly struggling with bloating. The allergies and mood swings I had when I was I was eating cooked food have also disappeared. Many people who have switched to a diet of raw food tell me that they're enjoying these same benefits from eating raw, in addition to others I haven't mentioned here.

Eating in the Raw included some easy-to-make recipes, but it was never intended to be a cookbook or a book of menus. I learned a long time ago that it is best not to overwhelm people with too much information on raw food at one time. The important things are to get them interested by explaining the benefits of eating raw food over cooked, to give them some encouragement and inspiration, and to show them what to do and how to do it. I knew what people needed because they are what I needed to get started. Still, once the book was published, people told me they wanted more recipes and more inspiration.

This book is the "more" those readers have been asking for.

■ ■ ■

Since *Eating in the Raw* was published, I have heard from all sorts of people who eat all kinds of cooked food about health issues, from headaches to asthma, allergies, dry skin, depression, brittle hair or loss of hair, high blood pressure, being overweight, suffering from heart disease and, yes, even cancer. I will often hear someone say, "I know you eat that way, but I can't go raw. I can't live on just vegetables. It must be horrible. I have to have my pasta."

Imagine the looks on their faces when I tell them that they can do just about anything they want to if they really want to do it. The truth is, of course, I eat a lot more than just vegetables. As for the famous carrots, I eat hardly any of them. But I do eat tiramisu, for example, and cookies, and pie and ice cream when I want to. They're all raw, of course, and guess what? They are just as tasty as the cooked versions that you eat—or try to avoid eating. And, by the way, my ice cream is more nutritious than your pasta, or the ham sandwich you had for lunch! I don't have any of the health problems that people who eat cooked food have—though I did before I ate raw food. So it's actually your choice if you want to continue eating unhealthy and being unhealthy.

In a world where nearly everything is cooked and processed, most of our experience of raw food is salad veggies. On the rare occasions when we eat raw food, it's as a small part of a cooked meal and not very appetizing by itself.

Whether we eat cooked food or raw, most of us eat more or less the same things from one day to the next, and this is especially true when we eat at home. Very few of us browse through gourmet cookbooks every day in search of a culinary adventure that will become tonight's dinner. Mostly we prepare our favorite tried-and-true dishes over and over again. These meals are usually simple to make and satisfying. If they weren't, we wouldn't make them repeatedly. Often people who are introduced to raw don't make the switch because moving away from these cooked staples seems too labor-intensive and it is tough to break a long-held habit.

With these thoughts in mind, what you will find here is a collection of 50 meals (the "raw 50" of the book's title) that can be made by anyone. The meals consist of ten breakfasts, ten lunches, ten dinners, ten drinks, and ten snacks. Some of the dishes are easier to make than others but they are all doable.

The breakfasts, lunches, and dinners include recipes that you might pull out and eat on their own—a soup or a salad, for example. Or maybe you're having people over and you intend to serve several desserts to your guests: select them from several different menus and try them out. There's something here for everyone and every taste. And for most of us there is enough of a selection in *The Raw 50* to start a list of raw staples that will never go stale.

My raw-food story is just one of many, and in *The Raw 50*, you'll find other testimonials that are even more exciting than mine. Most of these people don't live anywhere near the two meccas of raw foodism, New York and Los Angeles. While they may have been inspired by one or more of the well-known raw foodists, these raw converts haven't dropped out or run away to a raw retreat somewhere to live out their years as part of a fringe movement. They are real people leading real lives, just like you. I hope you will find their stories inspiring.

When I began eating raw, I knew hardly anyone else who had given up cooked food. Even when I started writing *Eating in the Raw,* my circle of raw-food friends and acquaintances was small. That has all changed now, and not just for me. The raw-food world is booming. So even if you don't live next door to someone else who eats raw, thanks to the Internet there's no longer a reason to feel isolated.

A few years ago it seemed the only way you could get the necessary equipment and ingredients to make raw food—from a high-quality blender to a vacuum-sealing system or even the ingredients themselves—was to live in a major city. Even in Manhattan, many health-food stores didn't stock a lot of raw-food items. Shopping meant making several stops at stores spread out all across town. Eating raw was hard, time-consuming work. That has all changed too.

■　■　■

By the time I wrote *Eating in the Raw,* the Internet had become a major source of information about raw food, and more and more companies that sold raw food were launching websites. Your ability to find what you wanted was no longer dependent on whether or not you had a Whole Foods supermarket in your hometown. The Nature's First Law site has long been a treasure trove for vegan raw-food products. Now there are more and more places online to get specialty items, such as gourmet raw cookies and crackers. And for those who are not strictly vegan, there are places to get a variety of raw cheeses and all sorts of other things as well. Thanks to the Internet, now you can find almost anything you want and have it shipped directly to you. Check out my website, Carolalt.com, too.

Thankfully, health-food stores everywhere are now stocking raw selections like never before. Even the major discount stores are beginning to get into the groove. Wal-Mart recently announced that it will add an organic produce section in each of its superstores, and Target now stocks some raw items. The major natural food store chains—Whole Foods and Wild Oats are the two largest—may not offer the best prices, but they are building and opening new stores every week. And there are more and more raw restaurants, cafes, and take-out places as well as juice bars sprouting up everywhere (no pun intended)!

In the "Raw 50 Staples" section, we've included a lot of helpful advice and info on starting your raw lifestyle, from outfitting a raw kitchen and stocking it with food, to the health benefits of raw staples and the decision to go vegan or not.

■ ■ ■

If *Eating in the Raw* is "a beginner's guide to getting slimmer, feeling healthier, and looking younger the raw-food way," think of *The Raw 50* as an essential hand-book for meals, snacks, and drinks. Even more important, think of it as your link to a community of people who have embarked on the same journey to a healthier, happier, and more fulfilled life. If you're afraid of giving up cooked food or still not certain—despite all its benefits—that raw food is for you, here are a few bits of advice from someone who at first feared going raw too.

- **Take it easy! Calm down, relax.** There is no reason to become anxious or fear-ful. This isn't a lobotomy or a stomach stapling you're agreeing to. There is no reason to be afraid!

- **Go slow.** Add a few raw items to your menu each day. Don't be afraid to try new things. You may not like everything. That's okay. Not everyone is going to like everything. And everyone likes different things. You will find the staples you like.

- **Be sure to eat a variety of foods.** Variety is the spice of life. It is also the best way to make sure you are getting the full range of nutrients your body needs.

- **Don't allow the people around you (who might feel threatened by the won-derful changes that are happening to you) to sabotage your progress.** Let me tell you that as you change the status quo, they will, absolutely, try to keep things as they have always been. Don't let other people control you!

- **Never be discouraged by your progress.** You're changing deeply rooted, life-long habits—ones that may be life threatening but have become a very real part of life for you—into new ones that may be lifesaving; that takes time!

- **Most important, don't try to measure your progress by anyone else's.** Not by mine, not by the other people's whose stories are in this book. Remember, we've had a head start! Join us, but measure your success by the changes in your own life.

Everyone's journey to raw is a personal one. Sure, it's great if you can become 100 percent raw, but even being 75 to 85 percent raw in the end will revolutionize your life. Give yourself time to try new things, to explore.

Now relax. Read this book. Think about what you like to eat now, and then do some investigating into where you can find the raw substitutes for those favorite foods. See how different eating raw is from all those worthless diets you have tried before.

Try it for thirty days and create a new habit of how to eat. See how different you feel and look. What have you got to lose besides some unwanted pounds, a few over-the-counter medications, and the poisonous toxins that are rampant in your body? And what do you stand to gain? Better health, energy, vitality, and youth!

Steal back your life starting right now! You're not alone. I and others like me are here to help!

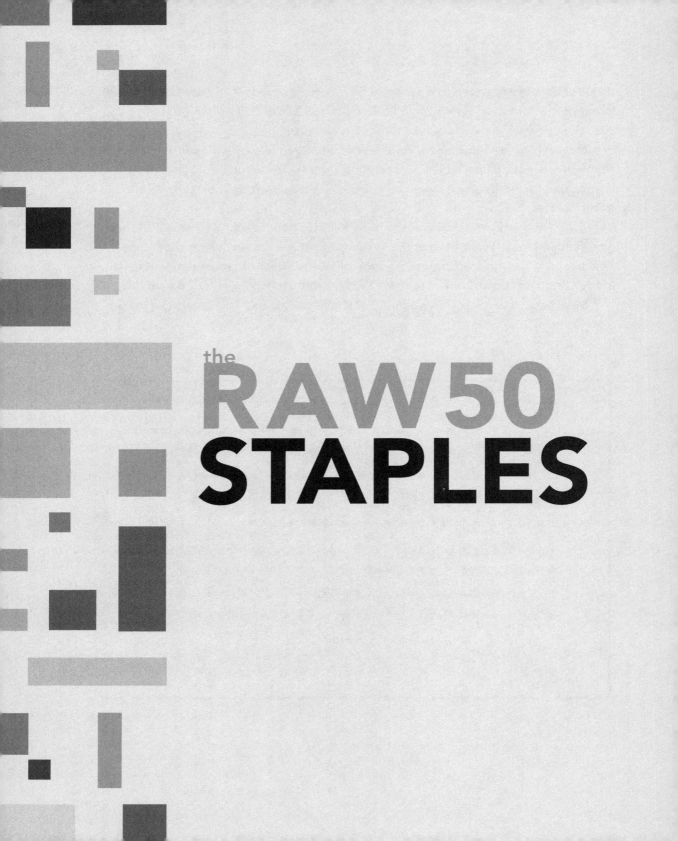

the
RAW50
STAPLES

Before I get to the recipes themselves, I want to outline the Raw 50 staples, and the steps you can take so you're ready to make raw meals. There is information on outfitting your raw kitchen and a raw staples shopping list. Certain easy raw skills are necessary, like sprouting and germinating seeds, and I go into them here. I also go through and describe commonly used raw ingredients like **raw dairy products, water, kefir, salt, natural sweeteners, miso, flax seeds, fruits, oils, and raw preserves** so you're all set up and good to go. I also give my personal answer to the question of whether or not to go vegan.

OUTFITTING THE RAW KITCHEN

I remember my mother's kitchen. There were pots and pans to cook in, lidded glass casserole dishes to use in the oven, and lots of Tupperware for leftovers. On the countertop was a toaster, right beside the blender.

Well, at least I still use a blender.

Over time, our kitchens become the place where all sorts of gizmos and gadgets accumulate. If you've been cooking for even a few years, look around your kitchen and you're sure to find appliances and utensils you rarely use, tucked away in a cabinet or taking up space on a countertop. Now is your chance to replace them with something new, something you'll actually use.

Doing away with cooking means doing away with many things: toasters, microwaves, even pots and pans. I use my stove to heat water for tea. I don't really need my oven at all. You may have a well-outfitted kitchen for cooking, but there are a few things you probably don't have that you'll want to invest in if you're going to be preparing your own raw food.

Here are the key pieces of equipment you'll need:

BLENDER

There are blenders, and then there are blenders. I remember the flimsy one my mother used, and I have destroyed many of my own over the years. But since blending is a cornerstone of raw-food preparation, you can't make a better investment than purchasing a nearly indestructible, top-notch blender. My favorite is the Vita-Mix.

JUICER

When I wrote *Eating in the Raw*, I didn't even own a juicer. My favorite drinks were the smoothies I made in my Vita-Mix and those I bought from the juice bars throughout New York City. At the time, I thought it was just easier to let someone else blend fruits and vegetables into sumptuous, savory, nutritious drinks. When I bought my juice at the juice bar, though, I had no choice but to drink it right away; juices start to oxidize as soon as they're exposed to air. In as little as twenty minutes they can lose most of their nutrition. It's a case of diminishing returns: the longer you wait to drink them, the less nutritious juices become. Having my own juicer would assure me of fresh, more nutritious juice right when I want it. But the juicers I had heard about and seen in use cost a small fortune!

Then I learned about Jack LaLanne Power Juicers. Now I'm hooked. This juicer does everything the $500 and $600 juicers do for less than $100, so this is an investment definitely worth making.

DEHYDRATOR

The dehydrator is to a raw foodist what the oven is to Betty Crocker. Yes, you can get by without one, but so many of the really incredible things you may want to make—from fresh fruit preserves to breads—call for a dehydrator. If you don't want to shell out for the versatile top-of-the-line Excalibur, buy a cheaper one with a reliable thermostat to start. Do look for some extra Teflex sheets too (in addition to the one that comes with your dehydrator). Teflex is a nonstick material used like wax paper, which keeps your dehydrating foods from dripping through the dehydrator shelves. A necessity when making preserves or cookies!

COFFEE GRINDER

No, this isn't so you can have fresh-ground coffee as you ponder *The Raw 50*. A blender as powerful as the Vita-Mix is too big for many small chopping or grinding jobs. Whether you're grinding nuts or a dry, raw cheese, the best and cheapest tool I know is an inexpensive electric coffee grinder.

INSTANT-READ THERMOMETER

Not everything raw has to be cold, but when you do warm food, you don't want it to get too hot. This handy device will help you keep things warm but less than 115 degrees F so that the enzymes won't be compromised.

SPIRAL SLICER

I said it once and I'll say it again: if there has ever been an appliance that is worth every cent, this is it! Spiral slicers (also called "spiralizers") are sold for as little as $20. Why is this such a handy tool? It takes vegetables and cuts them into a spiral shape that is perfect for special treats like raw pasta!

MANDOLINE

You can easily get by without one, but a mandoline slicer makes cutting vegetables into very thin slices easier and a lot faster than doing it by hand. They are available at a wide variety of price points.

VACUUM STORAGE SYSTEM (VACSY)

Unless you eat everything you make right away, this is an appliance you will definitely want to invest in. I couldn't live without my VacSy. Its glass containers are unique. They not only store food, but also, with the help of their small, handheld vacuum pump, allow you to suck the air out, creating an oxygen-free environment that preserves your leftovers.

OTHER ODDS AND ENDS

Most of the other accessories you'll need for your raw kitchen are likely already there. If you don't have canning jars and cheesecloth (or a stocking!) for germinating and sprouting, you should probably get some.

YOUR RAW STAPLES SHOPPING LIST

When I was growing up, you were sure to find milk, eggs, bread, sugar, flour, butter, and OJ in our kitchen as well as Tab, my mother's favorite soft drink, boxes of sugary breakfast cereal, and Oreo cookies. Today my shopping list looks very different, fortunately.

You have to cover the basics. And the sooner you get used to shopping for raw staples, the easier sticking to a raw diet becomes. Keep in mind that fresh, living foods naturally perish more quickly than cooked, processed ones, so shop for produce often and conservatively to avoid spoilage.

Most important, always remember to read labels. You want raw products, not their cooked counterparts. Labeling can be vague or even deceptive, and unless you see the word "raw" or an equivalent—"unpasteurized," or "cold-pressed," for example—chances are it is not raw. And always get organic if you can.

You should be able to get everything on the following pages at a natural foods supermarket such as Wild Oats or Whole Foods. For certain items you may need to visit a good health-food store or check out an online resource or my website, Carolalt.com. If you're vegan, you will skip some items on the list—honey, for example.

THE BASIC PANTRY

Refrigerator Section

Udo's Choice oil blend
(a cold-pressed seed mixture—tasty for salads!)

Raw milk

Raw-milk cheeses

Organic, fertile eggs

Dried Fruits, Legumes, and Nuts

Cashews

Almonds

Sunflower seeds

Macadamia nuts

Pine nuts

Flax seeds (dark and light)

Dates

Raisins

Dried lentils

Dried chickpeas

(Nuts can also be found in bulk, along with lentils and chickpeas, in stores that sell bulk foods, and at health-food stores.)

Miscellaneous

Cold-pressed, extra-virgin olive oil
("cold pressed" are the key words)

Agave nectar
(again, look for the word "raw" on the label)

Raw, virgin coconut oil and shredded coconut

Carob powder or raw chocolate nibs

Raw almond butter
(Be careful because several brands sell both raw and roasted under the same label; only the raw variety says RAW!)

Spices and Condiments

Bragg's raw apple cider vinegar

Bragg's Liquid Aminos

Nama Shoyu
(raw soy sauce)

Raw honey
(Look for the word "raw" on the label)

Himalayan salt
(evaporated, not iodized)

Sun-dried tomatoes

Cayenne pepper

Ground cinnamon

Cumin seeds and ground cumin

Dill

Frozen Foods

Manna bread
(This is cooked on the outside, but raw on the inside; available in carrot and raisin, cinnamon and date, fruit and nut, multigrain, and rye.)

Ezekiel 4:9 and Genesis 1:29 breads
(These are not raw, though they are made with all sprouted ingredients, but they are a good stepping-stone to sprouted raw breads.)

Organic frozen fruit with syrup
(for smoothies)

Fish/Meat Section

Spence and Co. gravlax
(Usually available at Whole Foods. Make sure you read the label; you want cured, not smoked fish!)

Proscuitto
(which is cured pork)

And in case are not making your own, don't forget:

Drinks

Water

Orange juice
(You want fresh-squeezed or the fully frozen, unpasteurized kind, not the frozen concentrates and not the "not-from-concentrate" pasteurized OJ in the dairy section.)

Herbal tea

Fresh Produce

Remember to get whatever is in season and whatever you know you'll eat. You'll find raw recipes often use:

Avocados

Bananas

Red, orange, and yellow bell peppers

Young coconuts
(not the hard, dark-shelled ones)

Onions

Garlic

Tomatoes

Lettuces and "spring mix"

Spinach

Lemons and limes

Oranges

Apples

Berries: blueberries, strawberries, raspberries

Mangos

Zucchini

Celery

Fresh herbs such as parsley, basil, rosemary, sage, cilantro (coriander)

Jalapeño peppers

Gingerroot

Remember; try to get organic if you can!

RAW DAIRY PRODUCTS

Have you ever wondered if small dairy farmers go down to the local supermarket to buy pasteurized milk? Guess what? They don't. They get theirs fresh from the source.

There was a time when pasteurizing dairy products, a process that involves heating them to between 175 and 212 degrees F, made sense. A hundred years ago we didn't have reliable refrigeration or affordable vacuum sealing to keep things from spoiling in transit. Those days are long past, but old habits die hard. Go into any supermarket and just about everything in the dairy section will have the word "pasteurized" on it—as if it's something to boast about. Not to me it isn't!

Those who make real dairy products take pride in the fact that their milk and cheeses still contain all the wonderful nutrients that God intended. Their enzymes are intact. They are real dairy and they are raw.

I love unpasteurized milk, but I don't stop there in my search for raw dairy foods. Supermarkets with large cheese selections often offer some raw cheeses. The person behind the counter should know which cheeses are made from raw milk. At Whole Foods, for example, there is usually someone who knows enough about cheeses to ask you if you want soft, medium, or hard cheese, and if you have a preference for cow's, goat's, or sheep's milk. Better yet, they will let you taste what they have.

If you like Manchego or Emmentaler cheese, for example, ask for "raw-milk" Manchego or Emmentaler.

Each state regulates the sale of raw dairy products differently. In some places you are not allowed to buy raw milk, yet across the state line it is readily available. In Pennsylvania, where raw dairy is legally available, you can find fresh raw milk and cream at many farm stands and health-food stores and raw-milk cheeses in supermarkets. But there is a restriction on unpasteurized butter, which must be sold "for animal consumption" only. Of course, the same sanitation standards are followed in making butter as in making cheese so, since I'm an animal, I don't hesitate to buy and consume fresh traditional, Mennonite-made butter. Obey your state laws and be careful who you buy from.

For raw foodists everywhere who want raw dairy products, the Internet is a Godsend. These days, you can get just about anything shipped overnight, and the high-quality standards that producers of organic, raw dairy products adhere to make these products quite safe. Still, if you can buy locally, do! If you can't, check on the Internet for sources of raw dairy products.

Two more things: The shelf life of raw dairy is relatively short, and it is important that the shipper use proper refrigeration methods during transport. Always buy raw dairy products from a retailer you trust, and observe expiration dates carefully. When you receive your raw dairy, always keep it refrigerated and tightly sealed for freshness. In fact, because it is exposure to air that causes dairy to spoil, I recommend always using a VacSy (see page 26) to store milk, cream, and cheese in the refrigerator.

KEFIR

Kefir means "feel good" in Turkish. With a name like that, it's hard to resist learning more about kefir.

Kefir is a cousin to yogurt. It is an ancient, cultured, enzyme-rich food that helps to balance your inner ecosystem, build immunity, and restore health.

If that sounds more like a medicine than a food, let me assure you it's as tasty as natural liquid yogurt. While offering your body the friendly probiotic bacteria you get from yogurt, it also provides several additional strains of the yeast your body needs. Yes, your body needs yeast to control and eliminate the destructive, pathogenic yeasts that are trying to make their home inside the mucus lining of your intestines. If you eat kefir regularly, the bacteria and yeasts combine symbiotically to replenish flora and boost your immune system.

Kefir can be made vegan style from young coconut, soy, or rice milk. Most people, however, use cow, sheep, or goat's milk. Because of the fermentation process, those who are lactose-intolerant usually have no problem with kefir, even if it is made from dairy. But check with your doctor if this is a concern.

It's possible to find ready-to-serve kefir in health-food stores, but homemade is really the best. It's simple to make. All you need is a live culture-starter kit or a chunk of kefir culture, called a "bud," which is really just a spoonful of already made kefir. (I got mine from a friend at a local Indian restaurant.) A bud remains living but dormant when frozen, so you can keep some in the freezer.

Stir at least 1 tablespoon of culture into 1 gallon of milk. (The milk does not have to be raw; the bacteria reconstitutes the milk, making even cooked milk healthier.) Then wrap the bowl in a towel and place it near a heat source that is no hotter then 110 degrees F. Wait 8 to 12 hours for fermentation to take place. Using a larger kefir bud speeds up the process, while a smaller bud takes longer.

There is no one way to make kefir, so long as the culture is kept alive. During the fermentation process, kefir will separate into soft clumps (curds) and thinner liquid (whey). If you want smooth, drinkable kefir, stop the process and consume it before it gets this far along, but if you want kefir "cheese," just give it some extra time.

Once you start making kefir, it will become a regular part of your diet. I love to make kefir because I am absolutely sure of the quality, and I can have it whenever I want it!

In the wintertime, I wrap kefir in towels and place it on or near the oil furnace in my house to keep it warm (but not cooked!) and to allow the kefir bacteria and cultures to multiply. In the summer, I leave it in the sun for the whole day. Either way, I keep an eye on it. When it gets to my favorite consistency, I put it in the refrigerator to stop the multiplying process. I mix kefir with granola, agave, or fruits, just as I would yogurt, but in my book, kefir is healthier!

RAW EGGS

In 1926, Julius Freed decided to start a business in Southern California. The concept was simple: sell fresh orange juice from a spot by the road with lots of traffic passing by. Freed enlisted the backing of a friend who agreed that fresh California orange juice by the glass would sell, but who also knew Freed needed a marketing hook. If there was something special, something different, about Julius's orange juice, it might bring people who couldn't get it elsewhere to his stand. Julius added some powdered sugar and a secret ingredient, and the first Orange Julius franchise was born.

What was the secret ingredient? A raw egg.

In recent years, to address concerns about salmonella, the Orange Julius folks changed the formula, eliminating the raw egg. But fact has been overtaken by fear when it comes to salmonella. In 2002 the US Department of Agriculture officially acknowledged that only 1 in 30,000 chicken eggs contain salmonella, and these figures are usually for commercially mass-produced eggs, not the safer, healthier ones from free-range, organically fed chickens.

Eggs are an amazingly compact, inexpensive source of high-quality protein. They are also a significant source of vitamin A, riboflavin, folic acid, vitamin B_6, vitamin B_{12}, choline, iron, calcium, phosphorous, and potassium. I understand that for many people the issues surrounding eating eggs are serious ones, and many people feel very strongly that it is wrong to eat any animal products. But strictly on a nutritional basis, it's hard to find a better food than raw fertilized organic eggs. You want fertilized eggs because after fertilization, the enzymes in the egg are released, helping to digest the concentrated yolk and releasing the nutrients (which would nourish the chick if the egg had developed into one). That is why fertilized eggs are easy to digest and nutritious. Several recipes in *The Raw 50* include them; decide for yourself if you wish to indulge!

SUGAR, AND OTHER SWEETENERS

I grew up eating lots of sugar. Back then, "pure cane sugar" was advertised as a healthy product, but many of us knew that the sugar in the sugar bowl made you fat, rotted your teeth, and made kids jumpy. There simply had to be substitute without those unwanted side effects.

Then along came saccharine, an artificial, sugar-free, calorie-free sweetener, as well as aspartame, Nutrasweet, and other artificial products designed to satisfy the human sweet tooth. Research has shown, however, that some of these substances are not only unnatural but also positively dangerous. So how can we please our sweet tooth in a more natural way?

When I started eating raw more than a decade ago, it was hard to find raw sweeteners. Of course, raw cane sugar was available in health-food stores. But "raw" cane sugar is neither truly raw nor nutritious. Fortunately, today there are several excellent raw sweeteners to choose from on the market.

Keep in mind that even organically grown, plant-based sweeteners are not really all that nutritious for your body. But if you wish to indulge occasionally, and who doesn't, it's worth choosing wisely.

Honey: Prized since antiquity and praised in the Bible, honey is nature's original sweetener. Most people aren't aware of how many varieties there are. If all you have known is the garden-variety, supermarket honey, you're in for a surprise. The range of flavors, colors, and textures of raw honey are amazing. Some honey is liquid and some is semisolid. If a recipe doesn't specify which type to use, the liquid type is always used. Whichever you choose, make sure the packaging says "raw." My favorite is orange blossom honey, followed by clover honey.

If you are keeping to a vegan diet, you may not want to use honey, but honey has health benefits that many raw foodists want, especially the antiallergy properties that help those with hay fever, for example.

Agave Nectar: In the last few years raw, organic agave nectar has become the plant-based sweetener of choice for most raw foodists. Extracted from a Mexican cactus plant, agave is a high-nutrient liquid that, like honey, comes in dark and light varieties. Because it is a syrup, it is often used like liquid honey.

I love raw agave nectar and can hardly remember what life was like before I started using it. It's a staple in my kitchen.

Stevia: Until agave nectar became readily available, most raw foodists used stevia for sweetening, and some still do. I just never developed a taste for it.

One or two of *The Raw 50* recipes call for stevia, also known as sweetleaf or sugarleaf. It comes in both liquid and powdered forms. Because the powder is 250 to 300 times sweeter by volume than table sugar, it reminds a lot of people of artificial sweeteners, and some describe it as having a bitter aftertaste. I think the flavor is less like sugar and more like Sweet'N Low.

Stevia is popular in Japan, and has been widely used as a sweetener there for more than thirty years, with no known or reported harmful effects on humans. But animal tests done with stevia have suggested there may be negative health effects. Proponents of stevia say the problems are not with the whole herb itself, but with stevia extracts and isolated compounds such as stevioside. That's why, most raw foodists who use stevia argue, you should use only the truly natural varieties, which are green or brown, and avoid the white, which may be processed.

In 1991 the FDA said, "Toxicological information on stevia is inadequate to demonstrate its safety." They allow stevia to be labeled and sold as a dietary supplement, but not as a food additive. Still, there are lingering, unanswered questions about stevia.

Date Sugar: Dates are delicious, and you'll find them in many recipes in this book. Date sugar is tasty as well, if you can find it, but almost all the date sugar you see is not raw. Like the cane sugar product Sugar in the Raw, which is less processed than white sugars but not raw at all, most date sugars are processed at high temperatures. If you can find a truly raw, granular date sugar, try it. If you can't find it, make it; that is the beauty of the dehydrator. You can substitute date sugar for regular sugar on a 1-to-1 ratio.

Yacon: Until very recently, the Andean root plant yacon was virtually unknown in the US and Canada. Now it seems to hold the promise as the "healthy raw sweetener of the future." Yacon's flavor is often compared to that of a melon or sweet apple. It is usually sold raw as a liquid, much like agave nectar, but its simple sugar (fructose, or sucrose and glucose) content is extremely low and supposedly indigestible, and therefore ideal for anyone who is diabetic or watching calories. It helps regulate intestinal flora and prevent constipation, improves calcium absorption, helps to lower cholesterol and triglycerides, and seems to boost the immune system. I substitute yacon in some of the recipes if I am "uncooking" for a friend who doesn't eat sugar.

Yacon won't make you fat, rot your teeth, or make the kids jumpy. Imagine a sweetener that is good for you! We sure have come a long way from "pure cane sugar."

SALT, SALT, AND MORE SALT

Salt is salt, right? Wrong.

The word "salt" is a catchall term for the chemical compound sodium chloride. But not all salts are the same.

With all the bad press that excess salt has received, it's easy to forget that we need salt. The body uses sodium for all sorts of things, from maintaining the electrolyte balance inside and outside cells to regulating sleep, from aiding digestion to fortifying the immune system. Salt is essential to good health.

The common white table salt that most of us grew up with certainly adds flavor to food and, apart from some specific additives (often iodine), it's usually chemically fairly pure. To whiten and purify salt, however, it's processed at very high temperatures. That's right, table salt is cooked, whether you cook it again or not.

Since I started eating raw, I have mostly used evaporated Celtic sea salt, which is unprocessed and natural. It is not an unnaturally bright white color and it's not pure sodium chloride either—which is a good thing. Gathered from pristine waters, Celtic sea salt includes naturally occurring essential minerals that are hard for your body to get elsewhere. Celtic sea salt is only about 84 percent sodium chloride—salty enough to awaken your taste buds, but structurally complex enough to provide your body the trace elements it needs as well.

There are other natural salts, each with its own merits, but recently, I switched to what is to me the ultimate salt, Himalayan salt. If Celtic sea salt is good for you, Himalayan salt is the best on earth and the best for you.

Himalayan salt comes from the remote Himalayan Mountains, which cover parts of six countries in Asia. It is pristinely free of environmental pollutants and contains more than eighty minerals and trace elements. It's the purest and yet the nutritionally most complex salt on earth. Once hard to get, it is now readily available. You may not find it on the shelf of your local supermarket, but you can get it in many health-food stores and, of course, at Carolalt.com. However, before adding any salt to your diet, always consult your doctor.

WHAT TO DO ABOUT WATER?

There is no life without water. Our bodies are made up mostly of water. So who would have thought that something so simple, so common, would be a complicated subject? Sadly, getting pure, healthy water into our bodies is not an easy task.

In the early 1990s, the media started to draw a lot of attention to the fact that most common tap water was not only full of chemical additives but sometimes full of nasty bacteria too. Sales of bottled water took off. Madison Avenue got involved in making the water you drink a personal fashion statement. Now bottled waters are as numerous on supermarket shelves as soft drinks.

Simply putting water in a bottle, though, doesn't make it healthy. Water "bottled at the source" doesn't mean it's pure; it simply means it didn't travel anywhere to get into the bottle. A recent study showed that the quality of bottled waters varies widely. There is little correlation between where the water comes from and how pure it is, and there is no correlation whatsoever between the cost of water and its purity.

Most bottled waters come in plastic bottles that leach toxins. So no matter how clean the water may have been at its source, by the time it gets from the plastic bottle into your body I feel it's too polluted.

Distilled water is good but, again, not in the plastic bottles you find at the supermarket. Most water is best when it has been filtered and purified by reverse osmosis, then stored in clean glass bottles until you use it. You can purify tap water yourself right at home, but the system you'll need in order to do it can be expensive, and if you don't maintain it properly, the water it produces may be as bad as, or worse than the bottled water in the store. So it's just another thing you have to pay attention to, something else to maintain, another responsibility in an already full life.

Do your best when it comes to buying (read labels) or making your own water by filtering or distilling it. Do what you can afford, because water is important. Sadly, what should be the simplest of concerns is actually a very complicated one.

P.S. I turned my water woes over to my friend Jim Artress of Custom Air and Water, who made me a system I could afford. Now that I don't haul in bottled water, I save so much money that the system has paid for itself.

FIBER

Raw foods not only provide the enzymes and essential nutrients your body needs but are also the best way to get fiber in your diet. But who cares about fiber? And what is fiber anyway?

Fiber is the indigestible part of the plant foods we eat that doesn't get used by the body for energy. Instead, nature has enabled your body to use it as a way to get rid of built-up gunk in your digestive system.

There are two kinds of fiber, insoluble and soluble. Insoluble fiber passes through our intestines largely intact. It prevents and relieves constipation, moves bulk through the intestines, dislodges built-up toxic waste in the colon, and can help reduce hemorrhoids. It also helps to control and balance the pH in your intestinal tract, changing it from acidic (not good) to more alkaline. This is believed to help prevent colon cancer by keeping microbes from producing cancerous substances.

Soluble fiber dissolves in water. It prevents cholesterol from recirculating and being reabsorbed into your bloodstream and instead carries the cholesterol out of your body through the stool. It speeds up the passage of toxins out of your system through the bowel, which reduces the ability of these toxins to recirculate back to the liver. Even earlier in the process, fiber prolongs the emptying of your stomach so that any sugar you eat is released gradually and absorbed more slowly. As a result, fiber can reduce diabetes and total cholesterol, especially the bad LDL cholesterol. It also helps to reduce the risk of heart disease, diverticular diseases, and possibly certain cancers, including colon cancer.

In simple language: the stuff you eat eventually ends up in your bloodstream and your intestines. You can have murky blood and a stopped-up colon, or you can have a clear, fresh bloodstream and a clean, healthy colon. Without much fiber you get the former; with it you get the latter.

Experts say not to worry about the ratio of soluble to insoluble fiber in your diet. In fact, those who eat a largely raw diet full of vegetables and fruits get plenty of both kinds of fiber. Excellent sources of fiber include nuts and seeds of all sorts, apples, bananas, blackberries, blueberries, carrots, cherries, coconut, dates, figs, grapefruit, kiwi, oranges, pears, raspberries, spinach, strawberries, and raisins and other dried fruits. Virtually any vegetable, fruit, nut, or seed you eat, especially if it's raw, will contribute to your fiber intake. When juicing, save the pulp—it is fiber; mix it in with other foods, so you don't waste the pulp from your fresh-squeezed orange juice. Oats of any kind, and especially raw oats, are not only an excellent bottlebrush for your colon but also the ultimate, proven cholesterol buster.

Most Americans who eat processed and cooked foods and few raw fruits and vegetables get less than half the fiber their bodies need, and some get even less than that. By eating raw you can be certain that you're getting what you need.

Flax Seeds: I had never heard of flax seeds before I started eating raw, and they may not be a fixture in your diet either—not yet. But as even a cursory look at *The Raw 50* will show, they play a big part in the raw-food diet, and for good reason. They are nutritious, tasty, and can be used in a variety of ways. Flax seeds

- Are an excellent source of high-quality protein

- Are rich in soluble fiber, clean the colon, and act as a very gentle, natural laxative

- Contain vitamins B_1, B_2, C, E, and carotene. The seeds also contain iron, zinc, and trace amounts of potassium, magnesium, phosphorus, and calcium

- Contain up to 100 times more of the phytonutrient lignin than buckwheat, rye, millet, oats, and soybeans. It appears that lignins flush excess estrogen out of the body, thereby reducing the likelihood of developing estrogen-linked cancers, such as breast cancer. Flax seeds also seem to reduce the incidence of colon cancer. Besides their tumor-inhibiting properties, lignins also have antibacterial, antifungal, and antiviral properties.

While most raw foodists, including me, eat the seeds whole after soaking them, grinding them releases the fullness of their hidden nutritional treasures. Flax seed oil contains essential omega-3 fatty acids (EFAs), which the body needs, especially if you're not getting them from fish. EFAs speed up the metabolism, and that means you burn more calories. And everyone knows what that means: you lose weight! Store flax-seed oil in dark containers to keep it from going rancid too quickly.

Flax seeds come in two colors, light yellow and dark reddish brown. The lighter colored ones tend to be more delicate in flavor, while the darker varieties are nuttier and stronger, but nutritionally they are similar.

THE TRUTH ABOUT COCONUT OIL

Pity the poor coconut. About forty years ago coconut oil got a bad reputation after some research claimed to link it to heart disease and high cholesterol levels. It turns out to be a classic case of either mistaken identity or guilt by association.

Here are the facts I have found: What is not mentioned about this research is that the study used hydrogenated coconut oil, not raw coconut oil! The process of hydrogenization creates toxic trans-fatty acids, or TFAs (also known as "trans fats"). These TFAs enter cell membranes in our bodies and block the use of essential fatty acids (EFAs) our bodies need (that's why they're called "essential"). The result is high cholesterol and heart disease.

Raw coconuts and raw coconut oil, however, contain no TFAs, none at all. In other words, real coconut oil was never the guilty culprit. It's the evil, twisted, chemically altered cousin, hydrogenized coconut oil, that ruined coconut oil's reputation for generations to come.

The truth is that the benefits of coconut oil (also known as coconut butter) are hard to exaggerate. It is cholesterol free. It contains the only fat that goes into the liver to use as energy rather than into the bloodstream. Coconut oil accelerates the metabolism, and may help people with ulcers, Crohn's disease, chronic fatigue, and irritable bowel syndrome. It may accelerate the healing of wounds and helps to clear up acne. And coconut oil contains caprylic acid and two other fatty acids that may fight candida yeast infections.

And here's a simple beauty tip: I alternate coconut oil with body lotions on my skin. If the skin is the largest organ in the body and absorbs into the body things you put on it, then I would rather absorb pure healthy coconut oil and chemical-free body lotions, both of which I feel will put up a protective barrier, preventing my skin from absorbing the pollution that lands on it from the air.

By the way, the dark brown, hard-shelled coconut you see in the store with the dry coconut meat inside is just a Thai coconut that has had the husk removed, thus allowing the shell to dry out and crack. These cracks let in air, which then causes the coconut meat to go rancid from oxidation and become hard from drying out. That is why you want Thai coconuts (also called "young coconuts") that are still wrapped in their white, barklike cocoon! This husk protects the shell and in turn the coconut milk and meat inside, keeping them fresh until the coconut is opened. (See page 97 on how to open coconuts.)

HOW TO MAKE RAW FRUIT PRESERVES

There's no need to cook fruit to make jam or jelly. Raw-fruit preserves are tastier than their cooked cousins and easier to make. Here's how:

Peel, seed, and slice your choice of fruit and put in the blender. Blend until it is liquefied (about 3 minutes, the smoother the better). Pour the liquid onto dehydrator trays lined with Teflex sheets and place in the dehydrator. Do not let the mixture rise above the edge of the shelf. Dry the fruit purée until it becomes leathery. This takes an average of 24 hours for drier fruits and 48 hours for juicier fruits.

Once the fruit has reached the desired texture, soak the fruit leather in purified water for 1 hour. Drain and put the rehydrated fruit in the bowl of a food processor. Blend the fruit into spreadable preserves, slowly adding a very small amount of water through the feed tube as needed.

Spread the preserve on your favorite raw, dehydrated cracker or unbaked bread.

TIP

Preserves can also be transformed into fruit syrup in the food processor. Gradually increase the amount of water added and whir in the blender until the consistency is that of syrup.

ONION AND GARLIC

Both onion and garlic are essential items in the raw pantry and both have many beneficial properties. Onions have antioxidant and anti-inflammatory properties and work to combat cholesterol and cancer. They are sometimes used to treat blisters and boils, and some products used in the treatment of scars contain onion extract.

Garlic was used as an antiseptic to prevent gangrene during both World Wars; it has antibacterial properties and is used in treatments for intestinal parasites. Garlic helps with fungal infections, digestive disorders, cardiovascular problems, cholesterol, and candidiasis (vaginal yeast infections are one indication of a candidiasis infection; moodiness and bloating are some others).

My father used garlic to reduce his high blood pressure and hypertension. Dr. Robert Marshall of Premier Research Labs in Austin Texas makes a wild garlic complex.

The flavor of both onion and garlic are stronger when raw, so use accordingly.

BRAGG LIQUID AMINO ACIDS

This flavor-enhancing condiment is a great replacement for soy or tamari sauces because, unlike them, it is unheated and unfermented. It is also gluten free, unlike soy sauce, which usually lists wheat as the second ingredient (salt is the first!). Bragg is full of amino acids, which are the building blocks of tissues and organs and very necessary to the raw foodist.

VEGAN OR NOT?

Many people in the raw food community are vegans, though not all.

What is a vegan exactly? Put simply, a vegan is someone who does not eat *any* animal products, including dairy and honey. Vegans are distinguished from vegetarians, who do not eat animal flesh, but may eat dairy and eggs.

The majority of vegans (and vegetarians) eat cooked food, although some do not. In fact, the most recognized names in the raw-food movement are vegan. Their reasons for not eating animal products include concerns about how safe uncooked meat may or may not be, respect for other sentient beings, a reluctance to contribute to the violence and disorder of the world, and specific health concerns.

Not everyone comes to raw food the same way, for the same reasons, or with the same values and goals. My experience has been that most people embrace a raw-food diet because they have a specific end result in mind, such as overcoming an illness or disease, or losing weight. Along the way, some of those people might adopt a vegan philosophy as well, while others, like myself, do not. Similarly, most people never become "totally raw."

It doesn't have to be a case of all or nothing when it comes to raw food. Eating raw is not necessarily about having a radical, philosophical, or ethical conversion experience. The journey may ultimately take some of them down that path, but it certainly doesn't have to.

I adopted a raw diet so I could prolong my career by eating natural foods that would nourish me and make me healthy both inside and out, while allowing me to enjoy a wide range of foods. My first book included recipes for raw-meat and raw-fish dishes. Dr. Nick Gonzalez, the Cornell-trained physician who wrote the foreword to this book, is a leading researcher in raw-food and raw-enzyme therapies. He explained that over time, different peoples adapted their diets to their local environments and ecosystems; so not all of us evolved in precisely the same manner. Today we tend to travel extensively and relocate all over the earth. This is a modern phenomenon, too new to really affect our adaptation to new environments or to assess the results it may or may not have on our health.

Although I and millions of other people from all over the globe make our home in New York City, our genetic roots are planted deeply elsewhere. People change location, but their roots will always remain their roots and may be planted somewhere thousands of miles, and many climates and cultures, away. We end up biologically adapting to different diets based on where we transplant ourselves. Yet for our bodies, our optimal diet and nutrition will always be based in our roots, which often are grounded in faraway places and environments we have lost track of and no longer identify with. In other words, what feeds me best may not be what best feeds my neighbor, like it or not. It seems that some of us evolved for optimal nourishment through eating meat or fish or dairy, while others of us did not.

I believe your body knows what it needs and will tell you. Although you may want to be vegan, you may find that your body is genetically adapted to animal products; you may even need them. On the other hand, you may feel wonderfully satisfied without animal products in your diet, and if that's so, my hat's off to you!

My advice is do the best you can, eat what you think you need and feel is right, and be patient and tolerant of others. And most important, check with your doctors when it comes to your diet.

SPROUTING AND GERMINATING

One reason raw foodists eat so many seeds, beans, and nuts is because they are not only versatile, but also veritable treasure troves of nutrition. Valuable as they may be, Mother Nature has seen to it that they are tightly locked. Fortunately for us, releasing their enzyme inhibitors and freeing their nutrients is simply a matter of immersing them in water, which can be done by germinating or sprouting. Seeds and beans can be germinated, and given more time they can be sprouted. Nuts germinate, but most will not sprout.

Most raw foodists take germinating for granted—it is something they do routinely, and it is essentially a once-and-you're-done deal: you soak, walk away, then come back and after rinsing, you can now use what you soaked and what has germinated in your absence. Sprouting takes a little more time, but is still a fairly simple process.

Unless they state otherwise, the recipes in this book assume that you are germinating all seeds, beans, and nuts.

Remember to use only dried, raw, and preferably organic seeds, beans, and nuts. Roasted, canned, jarred, or otherwise processed products (which, by definition, are cooked) will not germinate.

GERMINATING, STEP-BY-STEP

To begin the germination process, rinse the beans, nuts, or seeds; place them in a glass bowl or jar with under an inch of purified water; and soak them at room temperature for the amount of time indicated on the chart on the next page. Cover the glass jar or bowl with cheesecloth or a stocking to keep the bugs out.

After they have soaked for the appropriate amount of time, rinse and drain the germinated beans, nuts, or seeds with purified water a couple of times. They are now ready to eat or use in any recipe. They can also be dehydrated after germination for use in foods such as granola.

THE ONE, TWO, THREE OF SPROUTING

To turn germinated seeds or beans into sprouts

1. Put the germinated beans or seeds, such as chickpeas or almonds, in a sprouting container or bowl, making sure that they are well drained and well ventilated. Again, cover the container's open end with a fine mesh stocking or cheesecloth.

2. Set the sprouting container on your counter and allow the beans or seeds to sprout for the required time (see the chart opposite).

3. Rinse the sprouted nuts or seeds with purified water a couple of times for good measure, and drain well.

You can either eat your sprouts right away or store them for up to 5 or 6 days—after that point they are likely to become bitter. Always store sprouts in an airtight (not vacuum-sealed) container in your refrigerator.

GERMINATING AND SPROUTING TIMES

INGREDIENT	SOAKING TIME FOR GERMINATION	SPROUTING TIME
ALFALFA	8 hours	2–5 days
ALMONDS*	8–12 hours	12 hours
BARLEY	6 hours	3–4 days
BUCKWHEAT	6 hours	2 days
CASHEWS*	2–2½ hours	n/a
CHICKPEAS	12 hours	12 hours
KAMUT	7 hours	2–3 days
LENTILS	8 hours	12 hours
MUNG BEANS	1 day	2–5 days
MUSTARD	8 hours	2–7 days
NUTS (OTHER THAN ALMONDS, * CASHEW, AND WALNUTS)	6 hours	n/a
OAT GROATS	6 hours	2 days
PUMPKIN	8 hours	1 day
RADISH	8 hours	2–4 days
RED CLOVER	8 hours	2–5 days
RYE	8 hours	3 days
SESAME SEEDS	8 hours	1–2 days
SPELT	7 hours	2 days
SUNFLOWER SEEDS	2 hours	2–3 days
WALNUTS*	4 hours	n/a
WHEAT BERRIES	7 hours	2–2½ days
WILD RICE	9 hours	3–5 days

*Almonds are the only nuts that sprout easily. In fact, almonds are most nutritious when sprouted. Note that their sprouts will be very small, even after 12 hours of sprouting time.

10 RAW BREAKFASTS

What is a breakfast, anyway? When you think of breakfast, what comes to mind? For most Americans this "most important meal of the day" may mean a cup of coffee with sugar, accompanied by a bagel or a muffin. Or maybe it's cereal with milk; fried eggs with potatoes, bacon, and toast; pancakes with syrup; or yogurt and a glass of juice.

Outside of the Western world, breakfast choices are often more exotic: The Japanese sometimes start their day with poached salmon, rice, and a salad. (Maybe that is one reason why Japanese people, before they started adopting Western dietary practices, used to have such low rates of cancer and heart disease.)

Those who eat raw food—especially beginners— often turn to foods that look like their cooked counterpart whenever possible. That's why raw granola is popular. Even though raw and cooked granola look similar, the grains in your commercial cereal are, in fact, cooked. Under the intense heat, the grains are changed: the ratio of proteins to carbohydrates shifts in favor of carbohydrates. This makes your everyday cereal and granola a very sugary food. However, raw granola is germinated (see pages 41 to 43). Raw granola is reminiscent of cereal, but much healthier. Personally, I can't tell the difference by taste—only by how it makes me feel afterward!

Of course, you have so many options for how to eat your granola. You can pop it by the handful into your mouth, or if you have access to raw dairy, you can pour raw, unpasteurized milk over the granola. Or try some raw kefir (see page 30). If you don't consume animal products, you can always make raw almond milk to pour over your raw granola. Having choices is so important!

I like the expression "Eat breakfast like a king, lunch like a queen, and dinner like a pauper." To me that saying expresses the importance of breakfast over dinner. We need to start our day with a reserve of nutrients to carry us through. I have found that when I don't eat a great breakfast, I am hungry by eleven o'clock in the morning. If I eat a poor lunch, I am hungry again by four o'clock. And it seems I am not the only one, because sales of candy and snacks are soaring.

And while we are on the subject, who's to say we can't eat salad for breakfast? It's true that the standard American diet (funny that the acronym is SAD—how appropriate!) doesn't include salad in the morning, unless it's a fruit salad. But why not? No reason except we're not used to eating it that way!

Personally, I love a salad in the morning. Try an organic mesclun mix with cold-pressed olive oil, a little Himalayan sea salt, hummus, guacamole, and some crumbled cheese. The salad has all you need to carry you through your morning—and then some! I used to save some seared steak from dinner the night before (since you should eat a small dinner). I would cut it into pieces for my morning salad.

If I am on the run, a green drink gives me my salad in a glass! Or I will eat from a commercial raw snack bar. This sounds familiar, doesn't it? Raw food is no harder to manage than cooked. Stop kidding yourself, and start making yourself healthy!

Oh and by the way, if you are not a morning person, try making these dishes the night before and vacuum sealing and refrigerating them so that they are ready and waiting for you when you start your day!

One more thing: if you feel that you can't give up coffee, you might try to substituting Teccinno's roasted herbs for every other cup of coffee you drink. They come in several flavors: I like the vanilla, but you may prefer the mocha or coffee flavor.

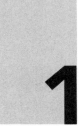

1 YUMMY, NUTTY RAW OATMEAL

SERVES 1

1 cup raw oats, germinated (see pages 41–43)

½ cup raw almonds, germinated (see pages 41–43)

¼ cup warm purified water (approx. 110 degrees F)

½ banana, sliced

Ground cinnamon to taste

Raw agave nectar to taste

The great thing about oatmeal is that it has been shown to lower cholesterol. The great thing about this oatmeal: I love it. And that's no mean feat. When I was a kid I never ate oatmeal, because I thought it was tasteless and gloppy. Looking back, I realize it was tasteless and gloppy. This oatmeal, on the other hand, is full of nuts and fruit and cinnamon, as well as oats that stand up under hot water and don't take on that unappetizing consistency I remember so well.

Rinse the germinated oats and almonds. Put them in the food processor and chop them coarsely. Transfer to a serving bowl, add the ¼ cup of warm water, and mix them together with a fork. Add the cinnamon and agave nectar. Top the oatmeal with sliced banana.

TIP

It can be a challenge to find truly raw oats. It's easier to find organic oats, but organic isn't the same as raw! Organic oats are still processed at high temperatures. Remember the rule of thumb is: Only if it says "raw" on the label is a product truly raw! Of course, you can always purchase your raw oats on Carolalt.com.

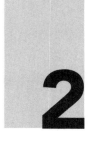

2 APPLES AND CREAM **MUESLI**

1 ripe Hass avocado

2 tablespoons fresh lemon juice

¼ cup raw liquid honey

4 apples, any variety

¼ cup raw rolled oats

¼ cup raisins

¼ cup raw pistachios, germinated (see pages 41–43)

Kelly's Macadamia Whipped Cream (optional, page 134)

TIP

If you think the muesli is just begging for more nuts, add more. Don't be afraid to add your own favorites, and feel free to toss in more fresh fruit too.

SERVES 1

I was at a friend's house in Switzerland looking for something to have for breakfast, when I found a box of muesli. I'd never heard of it before. My friend told me to try it—she loved the stuff—but to me it tasted like cardboard with little bits of fruit in it.

Now this recipe has very little in common with its distant Swiss cousin. It's called muesli, but it retains the flavor of all the individual ingredients. It also has oats in it, but it is creamier than the oatmeal on page 46.

Avocado tends to take on the flavor of whatever you pair with it—in this case honey, apples, and lemon juice. The lemon juice contributes a lip-smacking sweet-and-tart taste. Notice you don't need to use any water to make this dish. That's because the avocado becomes like a thick cream. Who in the world doesn't love cream?

Peel and pit the avocado and put in the blender along with the lemon juice and honey. Core and peel the apples, grate them to a medium or fine texture, and transfer to the blender. Add the rolled oats and raisins and blend until creamy, adding the pistachios toward the end to lightly chop them.

Spoon the muesli into a bowl and fold in Kelly's Macadamia Whipped Cream if desired.

3 YUMMY DAIRY MUESLI

4 tablespoons flax seed oil

2 tablespoons raw milk

1 teaspoon raw honey

3½ ounces kefir (see page 30)

2 tablespoons crushed or coarsely ground flax seeds

½ cup fresh seasonal berries or sliced fruit of your choice

Dash of cinnamon

SERVES 1

If you can find raw milk, I think you'll love this recipe. Many farm stores sell raw milk, but make sure it's organic.

Kefir is a yogurtlike milk product often found in Indian restaurants. I find it sweeter than yogurt. Kefir balances your system because it is probiotic. (See page 30 on kefir.)

This recipe is your substitute for the yogurt and cooked granola you may have eaten for breakfast, but it is even better, and, of course, better for you.

Combine 3 tablespoons of the oil, the milk, and the honey in a bowl and add the kefir gradually in small amounts. Put 2 tablespoons of crushed flax seeds in a cereal bowl, and cover it with the fruit. Top the muesli with the remaining tablespoon of flax seed oil and add a dash of cinnamon. Serve.

BREAKFAST TIP

No time to make muesli? Not a gourmet? Well, everyone needs a quick, easy breakfast for mornings when you are just too rushed to fix anything yourself. All you need is some granola made by a company called Good Stuff from Mom and Me, who have done all the hard work for you. The granola is raw, utterly delicious, and very healthy. It includes buckwheat, dates, sunflower seeds, raisins, almonds, pecans, walnuts, brown flax seeds, sesame seeds, and hazelnuts. All you have to do is buy the raw milk to eat it with. If you can't find raw milk, use a little almond milk. It's so quick and easy, your kids can help themselves while you sleep late.

This granola, and other Good Stuff, is available online.

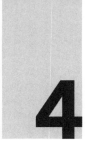

4 COMPLETE BREAKFAST SHAKE

1 ripe banana, sliced

½ fresh mango, peeled and sliced

¼ cup fresh pineapple, sliced

1 tablespoon coconut oil

1 tablespoon raw, smooth almond butter

1 tablespoon green powder

TIP

Mangos are a comfort food. Besides being rich in vitamins, minerals, and antioxidants, they have enzymes similar to papain, which is found in payayas and aids digestion.

SERVES 1

This shake is my sister Christine's favorite morning shake. I have to admit she did a great job with this recipe. The Complete Breakfast Shake is beautifully balanced, with fruit for flavor, banana for potassium, and, best of all, organic greens for nutrition hidden in the mix. That's pretty sneaky of my sister. Thanks to Christine, there's now no excuse for not getting your greens in the morning.

Combine the banana, mango, pineapple, coconut oil, almond butter, and green powder in a blender and puree until smooth. Pour the shake into a tall glass and serve.

If the shake is too thick for you, add a bit of water to achieve the consistency you like.

5 CASHEW BANANA SHAKE

¼ cup raw cashews, soaked for about 2 hours and drained

¼ ripe pitted and peeled avocado

2 ripe bananas, sliced

½ teaspoon raw vanilla extract (see Tip)

¼ teaspoon Himalayan salt

1 tablespoon raw agave nectar or raw honey

1 cup crushed ice

2 tablespoons raw cacao

TIP

The vanilla extract most of us grew up with is made with alcohol. If you have or have had an alcohol problem you may not want any alcohol, no matter how little. Those of you who follow Hilda Clark's teachings may not want alcohol because of its effects on the liver and because of possible parasites. If you want to make your own nonalcoholic vanilla extract, just steep a vanilla bean overnight in glycerine to cover.

SERVES 1

It took me some time to accept avocados in any recipe that wasn't guacamole. I didn't know what I was missing. Avocado tastes wonderful mixed with honey and banana. This shake is made by Raw Chef Dan Hoyt of Quintessence Restaurant. It's so creamy, you won't believe it. Before I tried it, I couldn't believe that avocados could taste so good, but now I'm a convert. I love this shake.

When you are ready for breakfast, blend the cashews, avocado, bananas, vanilla extract, salt, agave nectar or honey, and ice until they reach a milk-shake-like consistency. Pour the shake into a glass and serve. Add a little water (filtered and distilled if you have) to get the desired consistency, as this is one thick creamy shake!

Add the raw cacao for an extra boost. For me, it brings back childhood memories of chocolate milk.

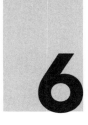

6 SIMPLE FAVORITE GREEN SMOOTHIE

1 head organic romaine lettuce, shredded

6 ripe bananas

TIP

Romaine lettuce is chock-full of nutrients. It is one of the best sources for vitamins A, C, B_1 and B_2, as well as folate, magnesium, potassium, and iron.

SERVES 4

I'm not kidding—Margi Ende's no-brainer smoothie is quite a surprise. My advice is, don't think about the individual ingredients. Just mix them up and go for it. I've made this smoothie in the past, intending to put half away for later, and ended up drinking the whole thing. It's refreshing and smooth and so simple and easy to make. What's more, it fills you up and provides the tremendous nutrition of raw greens. Margi's smart, no doubt about it. I wonder how many of her classmates at McMaster University start their day this way.

With the blender on a low speed, puree the lettuce and bananas, adding purified water as necessary for a smooth consistency. Pour the mixture into a glass and enjoy!

7 CAROL'S MORNING KEFIR DRINK

2 cups raw kefir
(see page 30)

2 tablespoon E3Live or
green powder

2 teaspoons coconut oil

2 tablespoon raw
agave nectar

TIP

My sister has found that
agave available online is
cheaper than store-bought.
Shop around for the best
source for your products.

SERVES 2

*This is my favorite morning drink. I make my own kefir so I can be
sure to have this drink every morning. The kefir is sweet, the
E3Live is nutritious, the coconut oil builds the immune system with
essential fatty acids, and the agave nectar is, well, agave nectar,
which is ambrosia from God. I crave this drink in the morning and
once I'm through with it, I feel so much stronger. Perhaps there
is one drink better than this, and that's the Mega Explosion on
page 53.*

Blend the kefir, E3Live or green powder, coconut oil, and
agave nectar thoroughly in the blender until smooth and
green in color throughout. Divide between two glasses
and serve.

8 CAROL'S MEGA HEALTH EXPLOSION DRINK

2 cups Carol's Morning Kefir Drink (opposite)

¼ teaspoon coral calcium

1 tablespoon colostrum powder

1 tablespoon Quantum whey protein

1 tablespoon Quantum-Rx Slim-Body whey

1 tablespoon tocotrienols

TIP

Don't freak out about the ingredients! You can find all of them at a well-stocked local health-food store.

SERVES 1

A friend of mine read this recipe and said, "Carol, I have to tell you, it sounds like a science project." That's not entirely unintentional. I'm throwing in this drink because nutritional science has helped us get what our body needs by making available in supplement form the best of raw foods and nutrients. But don't get me wrong. They're no replacement for eating Mother Nature's raw foods, but they can add potent nutrients to a diet of fresh, living foods. Think of this as Carol's Morning Kefir Drink with a punch for those mornings when you need an extra jolt of energy!

Combine all the ingredients in a blender and blend thoroughly. Pour the mixture into a glass and drink up!

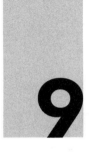

9 RAW GRANOLA WITH FRUIT

SERVES 1

GRANOLA

⅛ to ¼ cup raw rolled oats, soaked overnight and drained

¼ cup raw almonds, soaked overnight and drained

Small handful of raisins, preferably a mix of yellow and brown

⅓ cup dried cranberries

Seasonal berries or sliced fruit of your choice

Raw honey to taste

1 cup raw milk or Cheater's Almond Nut Milk (page 158)

A perfect, easy breakfast for one. When you see a food item described as "easy," it usually turns out to be anything but. Of course, companies just use the word to help them sell more products. But as far as this dish is concerned, I'm not selling anything other than the opportunity for you to have better health through amazing food. This really is easy—and raw and good for you. What else needs to be said? Nothing, except that it's lip-smacking good!

This granola and a glass of fresh-squeezed orange juice will have you looking forward to breakfast every day.

In a bowl, mix together the rolled oats, almonds, raisins, and cranberries. Top the mixture with your choice of fruit and drizzle with honey to taste. Add raw milk or Cheater's Almond Nut Milk if desired.

TIP

Drying fruit is easy. Buy organic when the price is right, and toss them in the dehydrator to dry them out before storing them. All you have to do is wash them, and depending on the fruit, peel them. For example, you may not want to eat a mango skin, but for blueberries or grapes you would.

This is a great way to enjoy seasonal fruits like blueberries and cranberries all year long. Most people never think about making their own raisins, but once you have tasted your own preserved grapes, you may never buy raisins again. Just remember, they take about 30 hours to dry, so make a big batch. When your family tastes these, they will go fast!

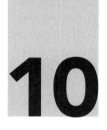

10 ALMOND RAISIN BREAKFAST COOKIES

1 cup golden flax seeds

1½ cups purified water

2 cups almonds, germinated (see pages 41–43)

25 pitted dates

1½ cups raisins or goji berries

TIP

No time to make cookies yourself at home? Miss Lillian's Oatmeal Raisin Cookies are made of organic oat groats, dates, raisins, apples, almonds, coconut, and spices. You can learn more about their creator, Harlem's own Lillian Butler of Raw Soul.

One Lucky Duck makes an oatmeal breakfast cookie too. It is sweetened with maple syrup (which is not raw, though the rest of the cookie is). Just the thought of it makes my mouth water.

MAKES 24 COOKIES

Who would have thought a model would offer you cookies for breakfast?

Okay, these aren't just any old cookies. They are made with germinated nuts and seeds, they are highly nutritious, and, of course, they are raw! Whether you eat them broken up in a bowl as if they were breakfast granola or as a cookie makes no matter. It's not the form, it's the function.

Soak the flax seeds in water for 1 hour or until all the water is soaked up. Put all the ingredients, except the raisins, in a food processor. Process until finely ground and well mixed. Add the raisins and pulse the food processor until the raisins are incorporated, but not ground up.

Spread a thin, even layer of the mixture on dehydrator trays lined with Teflex and place in the dehydrator. Set the dehydrator at 115 degrees F. Dehydrate for approximately 6 hours, or until the tops of the giant cookies are dry to the touch.

Remove the dehydrator trays, lift off the Teflex liners, and turn the cookies over. Place on the trays, Teflex side up. Peel away the Teflex liners. Place the trays back in dehydrator and continue to dehydrate for at least 10 more hours.

Remove the cookies from the dehydrator and cut each in half, and then each half into quarters.

Place the cookies back on the trays and return the trays to the dehydrator. Continue to dehydrate for at least another 14 to 15 hours, or until the desired consistency is achieved. The approximate total cooking time is at least 30 hours.

CHRISTINE ALT

Allergies and Arthritis
Long Island, New York

Siblings are notorious for being at odds with one other.

For more than ten years, since the day I began eating raw myself, I'd been urging my sister Christine to adopt my raw eating habits. No matter how much I tried to convince her to make the switch, she refused.

First, she said it was because she didn't want to get too thin. To be truthful, I understood. As perhaps the best and most famous plus-size model in the industry, she didn't want to do anything that would jeopardize her career. In the highly competitive world of modeling, that's certainly understandable.

But that wasn't her only reason. Christine also loved to cook and didn't want to give up her gourmet cooking to "eat carrots."

Deep inside, I knew that the day would come when Christine would decide she wanted to enjoy those same benefits that I'd discovered. Although it was hard sometimes, I decided to wait patiently for the moment when she was ready for me to help her change her life for the better.

One ordinary day in January 2006, I decided to stop in to see my sister at her home on Long Island. On my way, I picked up the phone and called her. "Don't come over," she said. "I can't move."

"What do you mean you can't move?"

"I am lying on my bed alternating hot and cold packs on my back and it's just not helping. I can't even get to the couch to sit and visit with you," she said, moaning in agony.

I simply couldn't believe my beautiful, vibrant, fun-loving, sister could be in so much pain that she couldn't live her life the way she always had, the way she wanted. So being the nosy sister that I am, I picked up my mom and went to see her anyway.

Sure enough, my kid sister was pale and looked like an old lady, not a beautiful model in the prime of her life. Not only was she in pain; she looked like a Old Master painting. Her skin was covered with little cracks that reflected light in every direction, like the cracks on the face of a Rembrandt.

Worse, she really couldn't move.

She told me she had been in physical therapy for three months, but instead of getting better, she was getting worse. And, she said, she had lost faith in her therapist, who seemed to be throwing up his hands in despair, not really knowing what to do to help her.

She told me she had three different problems with her back: a herniated disk, a degenerating disk, and arthritis. Quite a hat trick!

"Well," I thought, "God works in mysterious ways, and although I don't like to see my sister suffer to force a change, this is my chance!" I took a deep breath and told her I thought raw food might help her get better. Finally, probably out of desperation, she gave in.

I took Christine into New York to see my body therapist, Elizabeth Schoultz, Dipl. Ac., L. Ac. The first thing Elizabeth said to Christine was, "You are dehydrated." My sister's answer was predictable: "I drink a lot of water so that can't be," she said, proudly.

"She doesn't mean water," I said pointedly. Christine looked at me like I was crazy. I seized the moment. "She means essential fatty acids oils, more specifically, raw oils." Finally the lightbulb went on! Christine's look changed from confusion to curiosity, and I knew then that she was hooked!

Elizabeth worked on Christine's back for an hour and a half. When we were in the car on the way to her house, I gave Christine my "raw talk." I knew she'd be more inclined to listen now that she had a health problem or three. But since that was what had brought me to eating raw a decade earlier, I could hardly blame her. Why would she be any different from me—or from you?

I explained things to Christine the best way I knew how. I told her the body needs nutrients to make enzymes to digest food. The body does this because its most essential function on earth is to digest and utilize food and water. If you think about it, it's simple, common sense. Without food and water we die. Every other function of the body is secondary. Repairing itself, maintaining the immune system, even basic organ functions and elimination—everything else is a distant second!

The problem with cooked food is that it no longer has any enzymes of its own. So in order to digest cooked food, the body pulls nutrients from the most readily available source, itself. The body then produces enzymes to digest the cooked, nutrient-depleted food, which no longer has the nutrients to replace the nutrients in the body that were used to make the digestive enzymes. It's a big vicious cycle! As a result, the body begins to break down and age.

Here is an even easier way to look at it: To digest that cooked meal from last night, you will pull vitamin E from the collagen in your skin, resulting in wrinkles. You pull the copper that gives your veins and skin their elasticity, and over time this can lead not only to broken spider veins, but much worse, to burst veins in your heart (a heart attack) or brain (a stroke). And what about calcium? We all know about brittle bones and osteoporosis.

Those are just a few of the many vitamins and minerals we need every day. They not only make the enzymes necessary to digest food, but also help repair, rebuild, and maintain our bodies and provide a nutrient reserve for whatever else we may need in the future.

So, in a nutshell, cooking destroys essential enzymes. The body needs those enzymes and must re-create them when they are depleted for us sustain life. That causes a lot of stress and "dis-ease." Raw food puts back what our bodies desperately need, restoring biological harmony!

After the speech, I took Christine to Whole Foods for some raw staples. I showed her how to read labels so that she could recognize what's raw and what's not. Raw and cooked foods sit side by side on the shelf and usually look almost the same! In the end, it was more of an introductory lesson in raw-food shopping than a real shopping trip. When the cashier rang up the total, though, it came to more than $100. Christine was horrified.

Raw food isn't cheap, it's true, but it is far more nutritious! And you'll start to eat less food as your body comes back into balance and regains nutrients. I also assured Christine that there was a much bigger selection and better prices out there. I told her I'd show her where to get everything she could ever need or want, more cheaply and easily.

I had been doing a lot of my shopping at produce markets and through the Internet, but I knew I needed to make it simple for Christine and many others like her who needed some help. I wanted to KISS—"keep it simple, silly." That's why I started Carolalt.com. We are connected to almost everything. We keep an eye on the best prices, and best of all, we deliver everything right to your door. So much for excuses!

It didn't take long. Next thing I knew, I had a raw monster on my hands! Two weeks later I got a call.

"I am mad at you!"

"Uh-oh," I thought. "What did I do now?"

"After two weeks of raw, I have so much energy and I feel so good, but my back still hurts and I can't do anything with all this energy."

"Yet," I said.

"What?"

"Yet!" I said again. "Yet, you can't do anything, yet."

"So you mean I *will* be able to?" she asked hopefully.

"Give your body time to heal. It took you all these years to run your body down to this point. Give it time to repair and restore itself. Most important, don't give up. It will happen."

I am very happy to report that today Christine is not only running the wrong way up the escalators at the mall, but she is still raw, and she is making her own gourmet recipes, many of which appear in this book. She got her health back and didn't have to give up the cherished, gourmet side of her life (although she did have to give up a few unwanted pounds!). And not only is Chris's skin fresh and supple, and her back better, but she mentioned to me the other day that finally, after years of struggling with discomfort, bimonthly shots, and over-the-counter pills, her allergies are gone. No more allergies! No more! She is free!

As an added benefit, her husband, who is a regular Joe meat-and-potatoes kind of guy is not only happy with the huge changes in her vitality, her energy, and her health, but he even *enjoys* a few raw treats and raw meals himself.

"He saw major changes in me," Christine says. "He went from a skeptic to a supporter instantly!"

10 RAW LUNCHES

So, we've eaten our breakfast like a king. Next is lunch like a queen. I don't really know what it feels like to be a queen, but as the daughter of a New York City fireman who grew up on Long Island, I do know that I'm supposed to eat my lunch like one. And the following lunch menus provide midday meal choices that make me feel like royalty. I am sure they will do the same for you!

These are ten diverse lunches sure to satisfy the simple and adventurous palate alike. Choose something that fits your mood and allow yourself to take a break from the ordinary. And don't feel that you have to stick to the full menu. Mix them up. Pick and choose.

If you tend to eat at your desk in the office, it is easy to pack and store your meals. A simple plastic container can fit the bill, and the food should last unrefrigerated for a few hours. Nothing like "brown-bagging" it!

The same goes for the kids for school. Whatever happened to the lunch box, by the way? School lunches have come under scrutiny the last few years, and for good reason! Compared to a raw lunch, they are disastrous!

If you do decide to eat out at lunch, *Eating in the Raw* teaches you how to eat away from home and remain pretty much raw. Since I recommend that at least 75 percent or more of your daily food be raw, you have some leeway.

In case you don't have my first book, here are a few simple guidelines to help you along: Carry your own cold-pressed olive oil and Himalayan salt with you in a little plastic squeeze container. That way you are sure at least your oils and salt are raw. Order a salad and make your own dressing out of what you have carried with you. Then order a seared fish or steak and fresh fruit for dessert.

If you have eaten a proper breakfast, it will hold you until lunch and you should be able to resist the bread at the table and not be so hungry that you cannot order with your head. Don't fall victim to taking orders from your hungry stomach, which will call out for simple sugars. (See page 67 for my ideas on why wheat is not the best food for the body!)

Even though you may not be hungry at lunchtime, lunch is important. Skip it and you will be a four-o'clock casualty eating candy at a snack bar!

11 CHILI CHAMP LUNCH

Ingredients

1 cup raw pine nuts

1 cup pumpkin seeds

1 yellow bell pepper, seeded and diced

1 jalapeño pepper, seeded and minced

Juice of 2 limes

6 medium garlic cloves, 2 of them minced

¼ cup cold-pressed, extra-virgin olive oil

3 scallions, (white and green parts), chopped

1 teaspoon ground allspice

4 cups chopped ripe tomatoes

2 tomatillos, quartered

1 small fresh mango, chopped

1 teaspoon Himalayan salt

4 teaspoons chili powder

1½ teaspoons pumpkin pie spice

1½ teaspoons ground cumin

TIP

Don't germinate the nuts. Soaking the nuts in the marinade is sufficient.

SWEET MELISSA'S AUTUMN CHI-LEE

SERVES 8

I loved chili as a kid, but I'd get acid indigestion after eating it, which I now realize was the result of the cooked tomatoes burning my stomach. I can have all I want of this chi-lee, from Melissa Davison of Terra Bella Cafe in Redondo Beach, California, and I feel better after I eat it than I did before.

Chili lovers know that the varieties are endless. This one stands out, not only because it's not cooked, but also because it won a prize at the 2005 Texas Chili Cookoff in competition with conventional meat-and-beans chili.

Put the pine nuts, pumpkin seeds, bell pepper, jalapeño, lime juice, minced garlic cloves, extra-virgin olive oil, scallions, and allspice in a bowl. Stir together and marinate for at least 1 hour at room temperature.

While the first mixture is marinating, pulse the tomatoes, tomatillos, mango, salt, chili powder, pumpkin pie spice, the remaining 4 garlic cloves, and the cumin together in a food processor or blender. Transfer this mixture to another bowl and let it marinate for at least 1 hour.

Combine the two mixtures together and serve.

Variation: For a heartier chili, stir 2 to 3 cups of sprouted lentils into the first mixture before you marinate it.

LETTUCE SHELL TACOS

2 ripe avocados, pitted and peeled

2 tablespoons fresh lemon juice

1 medium Spanish onion

2 tablespoons chopped fresh parsley

1½ teaspoons ground cumin

1 garlic clove, pressed through a garlic press

⅔ cup sun-dried tomatoes, soaked and drained for 2 hours

1½ jalapeño peppers

½ teaspoon Himalayan salt

6 medium romaine lettuce leaves

SERVES 6

So this isn't a corn tortilla. But sometimes isn't it great to have the flavor you like and the lightness of body that you need?

I know P. F. Chang's restaurants offer stuffed lettuce wraps, and they sell like crazy. That many people can't be wrong. This is the raw version.

By the way, please don't be tempted to use iceberg lettuce. There is a whole book's-worth of reasons why I don't think iceberg is good for you.

Cut the avocado into bite-size chunks and sprinkle with the lemon juice. Chop the onion in the food processor, and then add the parsley, cumin, garlic, sun-dried tomatoes, jalapeños, and salt. Process the mixture until it is smooth and creamy.

Distribute the taco filling equally among the six lettuce leaves and then fold the ends of the lettuce together like a taco.

ZUCCHINI CRACKERS

½ cup golden flax seeds

¾ cup purified water

1 medium zucchini, cubed (approximately 2 cups)

2 cups raw walnuts, germinated (see pages 41–43)

2 tablespoons nutritional yeast (optional)

MAKES 24 CRACKERS

I can't eat chili without crackers or bread to slurp up the juices. In this book you have your choice of either—there are bread recipes in this book too. Mix and match as you like. I love to crumble crackers over my chili, just like my dad used to do. Be careful not to germinate the walnuts for too long or they will become a big pile of mush.

Grind the flax seeds in a spice or coffee grinder, and then transfer them to a bowl. Add the water and soak for about 1 hour, or until all the water is absorbed, stirring occasionally. Set aside.

Put the zucchini in a food processor and pulse until it is chopped into very small, uniform pieces, but not to the point of being mush. You want to retain some texture. Add the zucchini to the bowl containing the flax seeds. Put the walnuts in the food processor and pulse until they are finely ground, but again, not mushy or pastelike. Add the walnuts to the bowl with the flax seeds and zucchini and combine well (you may need to use your hands).

Once you have thoroughly mixed the ingredients, spread them out evenly on two dehydrator trays lined with Teflex sheets and dehydrate at 115 degrees F for about 6 hours. When the tops feel dry to the touch, flip the cracker sheets over on the dehydrator screens and remove the Teflex liners. Continue to dehydrate for another 3 hours. Then cut the crackers into the desired size and shape. Place them back in the dehydrator for another 11 hours, or until crisp. Serve with hummus, cheese, and guacamole; or with your favorite soup.

ALMOND
BANANA SHAKE

1 ripe banana sliced

1 cup almond milk

1 teaspoon ground cinnamon

TIP

For a creamier shake, freeze the banana slices first.

SERVES 1

Not full yet from your lunch? How about a beautiful banana shake with almonds? As Dr. Gonzalez notes in his foreword, germinated almonds may help protect against cancer. (They supposedly have estrogen blockers.) That is why I eat them and include them in every meal I can.

Blend the banana, almond milk, and cinnamon together in a blender until they reach a milk-shake-like consistency. Pour the shake into a glass and serve.

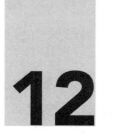

12 UN-SUPERSIZE ME MEAL

1 cup raw almonds, germi-
nated (see pages 41–43)

1 cup sunflower seeds, germinated (see pages 41–43)

6 celery stalks, finely
chopped

½ cup minced red onion

½ cup chopped fresh parsley

Juice of ½ lemon

Juice of ½ lime

1 garlic clove, squeezed
through a garlic press

3 tablespoons raw sesame
tahini

8 Sprouted Kamut Flatbread
Buns (recipe follows), split

Lettuce, sliced tomato, and
sliced onion for serving

Red Pepper Catsup (page
129), optional

Avocado Mayo (page 68) or
Raw Egg Mayonnaise (page
68), optional

TIP

To give your burgers a twist,
you can use quinoa instead
of kamut in this recipe, or
serve them on the Thyme
Bread (see recipe, page 98).

RAW BURGERS

MAKES 8 BURGERS

I gave up burgers when I found I couldn't digest the cooked meat any longer. And that was okay with me because I actually like raw burgers better. But I've always loved the process of making a hamburger and picking it up to eat it. This recipe gives me the perfect opportunity to do so.

Blend the almonds, sunflower seeds, celery, onion, parsley, lemon and lime juice, garlic, and tahini in a food processor or blender. Shape the mixture into 8 patties, and place them on Teflex-lined trays in the dehydrator. Dehydrate at 105 degrees F for 24 hours.

Place the burgers on the split sprouted flatbread buns and dress them with leaves of your favorite lettuce and slices of tomato and onion. Add one or two condiments, if desired.

SPROUTED KAMUT BUNS OR FLATBREAD

6 cups kamut, sprouted (see pages 41–43) (or use sprouted rye or buckwheat if you prefer)

½ cup plus 2 tablespoons raw liquid honey

¼ cup cold-pressed, extra-virgin olive oil

1 tablespoon Himalayan salt

MAKES **8** BUNS OR **16** PIECES OF BREAD

I can't help it. I love bread, but I know it's nonnutritious, fattening, allergy-forming, mucus-making, and bad for the body in just about every way I can think of. Have asthma? Well, how much bread or pasta do you eat? Everything has a cause and is a reaction to something, and in my experience, much of the time that something is wheat or wheat products.

This is where Raw Chef Dan Hoyt's kamut flatbread steps in. Like barley, spelt, or quinoa, kamut is a grain. This recipe may take a little time to master, but it is well worth it when you can stop taking your sinus meds. Why not make it a weekend project with your kids? Think about making a bunch of buns and freezing them or storing them in your VacSy system to keep them fresh. The VacSy will keep buns at least four days, provided you don't eat them first, and they can be frozen for longer storage.

After you taste these flatbreads and see what you have been missing, try to keep your thank-you notes to a minimum.

Combine the kamut, honey, extra-virgin olive oil, and salt in a bowl. Combine the mixture through a juicer with an optional mixer, or in a food processor, adding water if necessary. On a Teflex-lined dehydrator tray, shape the dough into ½-inch-thick buns or spread it about ¼ inch thick for flatbread. Dehydrate at 95 degrees F until the bread is dry, but still slightly soft. The buns should be dehydrated for 24 to 28 hours, flatbread for 16 to 24 hours.

avocado mayo MAKES 2 CUPS

"Hold the mayo?" No way! You can't have a burger without the works. Believe me, by eating raw, I don't want for anything. I can have the works anytime I like, and so can you. Choose between two different kinds of mayo. If you don't like this one, try the second recipe. I'll get you one way or the other.

1 cup raw pine nuts

1 large ripe avocado, pitted and peeled

1 tablespoon fresh lemon juice

2 tablespoons raw apple cider vinegar

1 teaspoon Himalayan salt

3 medium pitted dates

Soak the pine nuts in purified water for 6 or more hours. When the pine nuts have finished soaking, you will notice they have gotten plump with the water and are soft to the touch. Drain and rinse the pine nuts, then chop them in the food processor. Add the avocado, lemon juice, apple cider vinegar, salt, and dates. Process the ingredients together until creamy. Use the mayo as a decadent spread for raw burgers and store the remainder in a VacSy container in the fridge, where it should keep for 4 or 5 days.

raw egg mayonnaise MAKES ABOUT 1½ CUPS

Kudos to Brooklynite turned Southern Californian Tracey Oddo—this raw mayo with herbs makes a great dip for raw veggies or a spread for raw crackers! After trying this, you'll never look at its cooked counterpart again.

1½ tablespoons fresh lemon juice

1 whole egg, plus 1 egg yolk at room temperature

¼ teaspoon white or cayenne pepper

¼ teaspoon Himalayan salt

Additional dried organic herbs and spices of your choice (such as dry mustard)

1 cup cold-pressed, extra-virgin olive oil

Combine the lemon juice, egg and yolk, pepper, salt, and any additional dried herbs or spices you may wish to use in a blender and blend slightly. Then with the blender on low speed, slowly add the olive oil in a very thin stream until you have achieved the desired consistency.

MARTIN'S FAVORITE COLESLAW

1 cup shredded red cabbage

1 cup shredded green cabbage

½ carrot, shredded

¼ cup shredded yellow onion

1 tablespoon cumin seeds

Juice of 1 lemon

1 teaspoon Himalayan salt

2 garlic cloves, minced

1 teaspoon ground cumin

⅓ cup cold-pressed, extra-virgin olive oil

Drizzle of raw cider vinegar

1 medium tomato, diced (optional)

SERVES 4

Picnic time! You can't have a picnic with hamburgers without coleslaw. I put some right on my burger. This recipe is all raw yet it's just like a regular coleslaw recipe, and maybe even easier!

When David was working on the first book with me, we were experimenting with recipes. David's son Martin came up with this recipe, and not only did he love it, we loved it, too!

Put all of the ingredients in a large bowl. Toss to combine and serve!

YUMMY CHOCO-COCO **MOUSSE**

SERVES **4**

1 ripe Hass avocado (preferably without brown spots)

3 to 4 tablespoons raw agave nectar

1 to 2 teaspoons vanilla extract

2 to 3 tablespoons "Yummy" Coconut Butter

30 drops raw wild propolis extract

1 tablespoon fresh coconut meat (optional)

4 to 5 teaspoons raw cacao powder

2 tablespoons "Yummy" Tocos powder

⅛ teaspoon Himalayan salt

Raspberries, blueberries, or other topping, for garnish

My friend Christopher Dobrowolski has a great store called "live live and organic" on the Lower East Side of New York. Though he sells all sorts of raw-related products, Christopher has made a name for himself with his live live (that's the word live with a short "i", followed by live with a long "i") lines of body, skin and beauty care products, superfoods, and nonsynthetic supplements.

I'm always learning new things about the benefits of eating raw foods. Christopher told me these things about the ingredients of his mousse: Avocados are great for the brain, energy, and skin. Cacao powder in the raw form is rich in antioxidants, iron, and magnesium, and is a mood and energy elevator. Coconut butter is a good antibacterial agent and is antifungal. It is also a good source of hormonal support and increases metabolism and cellular energy. "Tocos" are really tocotrinols, a good antioxidant which is 30 times more potent than vitamin E, helps to lower cholesterol, and is great for the skin! Wild propolis seems to be the best overall natural immune system booster, acts as a preservative, and enhances flavor. Celtic sea salt contains a wide array of minerals and trace minerals, enhances flavor, and helps in digestion. Wow! All that in chocolate mousse!

Cut the avocado in half, remove the pit, scoop out the meat, and place it in a blender. While whirring, add the agave, vanilla, coconut butter, propolis, coconut meat, cacao powder, tocos, and salt. Blend thoroughly for a few minutes until smooth. Scoop mousse into individual serving cups and garnish with fresh raspberries, blueberries, or your favorite toppings. Serve chilled or at room temperature.

13 ASIAN PERSUASION LUNCH

1 fennel bulb

1 bunch fresh dill

1 scallion

1 jalapeño or red Thai chile pepper, stemmed and seeded, or 1 teaspoon red curry paste

⅓ small red onion

Juice and meat of 1 young coconut

5 fresh basil leaves

¼ pound raw cashews, germinated (see pages 41–43)

1½ teaspoons Himalayan salt

1½ teaspoons ground coriander

2 pitted dates

1 apple, preferably Gala, diced

1 avocado, pitted, peeled and diced

Up to 2 cups purified water

1 small bunch fresh chives, chopped or left whole

TIP

Coriander is the spice made from the seeds of the herb known by its Spanish name, cilantro.

ASIAN ANISE SOUP

SERVES 4

Can't go through a cold winter's day without something hot? I found that a hot soup makes me sweat for about five to ten minutes, but a hearty raw one like this Janice Innella creation, with all the right ingredients, sticks to the bones, filling me up and keeping me warm inside all afternoon. It's also a great way to get your daily dose of essential raw oils. It's the oils that will keep you warm as they burn off cleanly, and they also give you a beautiful glow! No wonder people call Janice "The Beauty Chef."

This soup is full of wonderful herbs. Fennel is excellent for digestion, where beauty starts. Dill increases the flow of a mother's milk after giving birth, and is used to treat bad breath, heartburn, colic, gas, and amenorrhea (abnormal menstruation). Anise is used as a natural treatment for asthma, bad breath, breast-feeding problems, colds, coughs, erectile dysfunction, female estrogenetic sexual problems, and sore throat.

Roughly chop the fennel, dill, scallion, chile, onion, and coconut. Put in the blender with the basil, cashews, salt, coriander, dates, and all but ¼ cup of the apple and avocado. Blend, adding the water as needed, until you have a smooth and creamy soup. Divide the soup among four bowls and garnish with the reserved apple and avocado, and the chives. Chill the soup lightly, or serve at room temperature.

NAMA SHOYU CARROT CRACKERS

MAKES 24 LARGE CRACKERS

I can't eat soup without some crunchies in it, and this is the perfect crunch as far as I'm concerned. Unlike most things, these crackers can sit in the refrigerator for at least 2 weeks. So when you make 'em, make a bunch to keep on hand. These crackers are great alone or with raw avocado mayo, humus, guacamole, or raw milk cheese.

2 cups dark flax seeds

3 cups purified water, plus a little extra as needed

2 cups carrot pulp (reserved from when you make carrot juice)

½ cup Nama Shoyu

½ cup Bragg Liquid Aminos

1 small garlic clove, minced

TIP

If you do not make carrot juice or have a juicer, you can finely chop the carrots in a food processor and squeezed them out in a clean old towel to dry them out.

Put the flax seeds in a spice or coffee grinder and grind well. Soak the ground flax in the 3 cups of water for at least 1 hour, or until all the water is absorbed. Put the soaked flax seeds, carrot pulp, Nama Shoyu, Bragg Liquid Aminos, and minced garlic in a food processor and process, slowly adding extra water if needed: the drier your carrot pulp is, the more water you will need. If your pulp is very wet, you may not need water at all. The mixture should be moist, but not runny.

Spread the cracker mixture on Teflex-lined dehydrator trays as thinly as you can without leaving any holes. Dehydrate at 115 degrees F for approximately 6 hours, or until the tops are dry to the touch. Flip the giant crackers over onto the dehydrator screens and peel off the Teflex liners. Return the crackers to the dehydrator for approximately 3 hours, or until the tops are a bit drier. Remove and cut the sheets into small, cracker-size squares. Place the crackers back in dehydrator until they are crispy and crunchy, approximately 6 to 10 more hours.

MURIEL'S DOUBLE-DUO DILL 'N' CUCUMBER SALAD

5 cucumbers, peeled and thinly sliced

2 tablespoons Himalayan salt

2 tablespoons raw apple cider vinegar

2 tablespoons cold-pressed olive oil

1 bunch dill, chopped

½ onion, chopped (optional)

SERVES 6

When I was a kid, my mother used to make a dill cucumber salad, mostly for picnics or barbecues, and the Alt family could never get enough of it. I wondered what made the salad so irresistible, so I asked my mom. She told me that the secret was pressing the cucumbers to "get the burps out." I'm not sure I know what that means, but to get it right, follow her directions carefully. This is a great salad. Thanks again, Mom!

Place the cucumbers in a bowl, add the salt, and toss. Place a small dish on top of the cucumbers and place a weight on top of that—a blender filled with water will do—to press down on the cucumbers, squeezing them for at least 2 hours. Then drain off the liquid, and take the time to squeeze more juice out of the cucumbers by hand. Discard the liquid. Place the cucumbers back in the bowl and add the raw apple cider vinegar, olive oil, dill, and onion, if you wish.

Mix well and serve the salad in one giant bowl. Let everyone enjoy it family-style!

Variation: Here is an easy "double" version of the Dill 'n' Cucumber Salad for those who like it creamy. Just make some Avocado Mayo (see page 68) or the Raw Egg Mayonnaise (see page 68) and add dill to it. Mix it with my mom's recipe, to taste. Now you have two cucumber salads, creamy and plain.

FRESH FRUTTA DI STAGIONE

Sliced seasonal fruit of your choice

Real-Dairy Whipped Cream (recipe follows) or Kelly's Macadamia Whipped Cream (page 134)

SERVES AS MANY AS YOU LIKE

One day my boyfriend, Alexei, and I were shopping at the local organic produce market. Alexei asked me, "How are these seedless grapes organic?" When I replied, "Well, they're grown without using pesticides," he gave me a quizzical look. He's Russian and speaks English as a second language, so at first I thought maybe he didn't understand me. Then I realized he was on to something. Obviously grapes are not found seedless in nature! They must have been genetically modified to be without seeds.

Organic means simple, healthful, and close to nature. How can something that should have seeds but now doesn't be considered "close to nature"? It can't. Admittedly, seedless hybrid fruits are not always genetically engineered in a laboratory, irradiated, or chemically altered. Nonetheless, I prefer not to buy anything seedless. While you'll find seedless watermelon and other seedless fruits labeled "organic," technically they're not, even if they are grown without pesticides.

Cut up your choice of fruit and serve in a bowl or parfait glass. Top with either Real-Dairy Whipped Cream or Kelly's Macadamia Whipped Cream.

real-dairy whipped cream MAKES ABOUT 1 CUP

I love, love, love whipped cream. I used to say that my arms grew longer whenever there was a bowl around. I could reach that bowl from anywhere in the room without getting up. At the same time, I understood all the problems with pasteurized cream, the least of which is that I was and still am a model and need to keep my weight down.

I don't have these same thoughts about raw cream. I don't get the same unhealthy reactions. I don't feel full. I don't feel fat. I don't get sinus problems or mucus congestion as badly. I'll never go back to pasteurized cream. If you can't find real raw cream but you need your whipped cream fix, don't worry. We have vegan-style, nondairy whipped creams made without any hydrolyzed or trans-fatty acids. (See recipe on page 134.)

½ cup raw heavy cream, well chilled   ¼ teaspoon vanilla extract

1½ teaspoons raw agave nectar

Put the mixing bowl and the beaters from your electric mixer in the refrigerator until they are very well chilled, about 20 minutes. Begin beating the raw cream with the mixer on low speed, gradually increasing the speed to high as the cream thickens, and continue beating until the cream forms soft peaks. Add the agave nectar and vanilla extract and beat briefly. Serve immediately, or cover and refrigerate for up to 2 hours before serving.

TIP

Be careful not to overbeat or the cream will become sweet butter—which, come to think of it, isn't too shabby in itself!

14 REAL MEN EAT RAW LUNCH

BRUCE WEINSTEIN'S SPINACH QUICHE

FILLING

9 ounces raw cashews, germinated (see pages 41–43)

½ cup plus 2 tablespoons water

2 tablespoons plus 1 teaspoon fresh lemon juice

11 ounces spinach, stems removed

1½ teaspoons dried parsley

1⅓ onions, minced

⅜ teaspoon Himalayan salt

⅜ teaspoon black pepper

¼ teaspoon white pepper

Pinch of ground allspice

4 apple pectin capsules

½ pound walnuts or pecans, soaked for 4 hours, drained, and dehydrated, at 105 degrees F for 24 to 36 hours

SERVES 6

When chef Bruce Weinstein chose the name Awesome Foods for his premade raw foods company, he chose well. I find regular cooked quiches heavy and buttery, and I don't like their greasy aftertaste. But this quiche is light and tasted so good that we had to call Bruce and ask him to honor us with his recipe for this book. It's truly awesome.

Be careful not to germinate the cashews for too long—they break down fast.

Grind the cashews in a food processor, adding water and lemon juice as you go to make a cream. Continue processing until the cashews have formed a smooth paste. Add the spinach, parsley, onion, salt, black and white pepper, allspice, and apple pectin; process again until smooth. Transfer the filling to a large bowl and set aside.

Grind the walnuts or pecans in the food processor until they are finely chopped, but not powdered. Press them evenly into a 9-inch pie plate to form a crust. Add the filling to the crust, distributing it evenly. Cover and refrigerate the quiche overnight to set. Serve it cold, at room temperature, or warmed (but never more than 115 degrees F).

RED LEAF SALAD WITH ARUGULA PESTO DRESSING

2 cups packed arugula leaves

½ cup raw pine nuts, germinated (see pages 41–43)

1 garlic clove, minced

1 teaspoon Himalayan salt

¼ to ⅓ cup cold-pressed, extra-virgin olive oil

3 cups torn red leaf lettuce

TIP

I used to eat salads as a snack when I was a kid, thinking that it was a good low-calorie choice. Little did I know that salad with bottled dressing was almost as fattening as a hamburger and fries! So be sure to make your own dressing—you'll find easy recipes on pages 116 and 124.

SERVES 2

When I first started to eat raw, I told Dr. Timothy Brantley I didn't eat salads because they didn't fill me up. Those heavy cooked commercial dressings, which are full of all the wrong kinds of fats, felt like a lot of empty calories because I was hungry an hour after I ate. Dr. Brantley asked me if I ate iceberg lettuce, which I did. He explained that dark green lettuce was a better choice, and he was right! Once I eliminated iceberg and opted for romaine, butter lettuce, spinach, and a mesclun mix, salad became a staple in my diet. As you'll see from this book, there's no shortage of interesting salad ideas. Don't be afraid to experiment with different salads and dressings from this book. Or make your own signature dressing. Have fun. Food should be an adventure and we shouldn't get stuck in a rut.

Put the arugula, pine nuts, garlic, and salt in a blender. Blend the ingredients together while slowly adding the olive oil in a stream until you have a thick dressing. Be careful not to add too much oil! To serve, divide the lettuce between two bowls, let each diner add some dressing and toss.

LEMON GINGER
COCONUT TART

FILLING

½ cup coconut butter

1 cup fresh meat from a young coconut, plus extra for garnish if desired

½ cup chopped fresh ginger-root

1 cup pitted dates

1 cup raw almonds, soaked for 8 to 12 hours and drained

¼ cup grated lemon zest

1 cup fresh lemon juice (about 4 to 6 lemons)

CRUST

2 cups raw almonds, soaked for 8 hours and drained, plus extra (do not soak) for garnish if desired

1 cup dates, soaked in warm water for 2 hours and drained

3 tablespoons ground flax seed

8 fresh mint leaves for garnish (optional)

SERVES 8

Once you've made Santa Fe–based raw chef Cassandra Durham's tart, trust me, you will be hooked. Her crust rivals the best baked crust out there. You can fill it with almost anything you like—fruit jellies or nut creams, for example. But ginger is so good for the stomach; it settles it down. And raw coconut? I cannot say enough good things about it. I love raw virgin coconut oil so much that I often rub it on my skin—all over! Just ask any makeup artist who has worked with me about my skin.

Dr. Gonzalez's advice is to eat ten germinated almonds a day to help prevent cancer. This is one fun way to get your medicine.

For the filling, scoop the coconut butter into a glass measuring cup. Immerse it in hot, but not boiling, water to gently melt. In a food processor, finely blend the coconut meat, gingerroot, dates, and almonds together. Add the lemon zest, lemon juice, and coconut oil and continue to blend until you have a creamy filling. Transfer the filling to a bowl and set it aside.

For the crust, combine the almonds, dates, and flax seeds in the food processor and blend until creamy. Pour into a 9-inch pie pan, tart pan with a removable bottom, or a cake pan. Use your fingers to form the sides and bottom of the crust. Spread the tart filling over the crust. Garnish with almonds, mint leaves, and strips of coconut meat as desired. Dehydrate the tart at 110 degrees F until firm but not complete dry, about 6 hours. Refrigerate for 2 hours, and then serve.

15 INDIAN DREAM LUNCH

RED PEPPER CURRY SOUP

3 bell peppers of your choice (red, green, or yellow), seeded and chopped

1 apple, peeled and cut into eighths

1 ripe avocado pitted, peeled, and diced

½ cup fresh basil leaves, chopped, plus 6 whole leaves for garnish

1 cup raw pine nuts

⅓ red onion, chopped

1 garlic clove, chopped

3 tablespoons curry powder

1 dried red chile pepper, chopped

1 teaspoon Himalayan salt

2 cups purified water

SERVES 6

I have already told you how I feel about Janice Innella's soups (see page 71) and this one is no exception. I spent a couple of months in India shooting a movie, and I got hooked on curry. If you love curry like I do, then this is the soup for you.

Set aside ½ cup of chopped pepper, 2 apples sections, and half the avocado for garnish. Combine the remaining pepper, apple, avocado, and the basil, pine nuts, onion, garlic, curry powder, chile pepper, and salt in a blender and whir to combine. Add the purified water and blend until creamy.

Divide the soup evenly among six bowls and garnish with the reserved pepper, apple, and avocado, and a whole basil leaf. Serve at room temperature.

TIP

Apples are an excellent source of vitamin C, pectin, fiber, lutein, and boron. They are also full of antioxidants that slow aging and protect against cardiovascular disease and cancers. (It seems it's true what they say about keeping the doctor away!) And with so many varieties to choose from, there is no reason to limit yourself to one a day.

SIMPLE FLAX SEED
CRACKERS

1 cup flax seeds, any type

½ teaspoon Himalayan salt

MAKES 12

No soup is complete without crackers, but these crackers are different—they are so healthy for you, it is ridiculous. There's no need to suffer to get your fill of flax. Eat these crackers in soup, on your salad, or with raw-milk cheese. Why are you waiting to do something good and healthy for your body? The answer is right in front of your nose.

Put the flax seeds in a glass bowl, and pour just enough purified water over the seeds to cover them. Soak them for at least 1 hour. After the seeds have soaked, without draining, add the salt.

Spread the mixture on Teflex-lined dehydrator trays so it is ¼ inch thick. Dehydrate at 95 to 105 degrees F for 24 hours or until crispy. Using a spatula, flip the partially dehydrated cracker sheets over halfway through the dehydration time, or at the point that they are dry on top. This helps to dehydrate the crackers evenly in less time. The crackers will shrink as they dehydrate. Break the sheet of crackers into pieces to serve.

SPINACH STRAWBERRY SALAD WITH RASPBERRY DRESSING

3 cups baby spinach leaves

10 fresh strawberries, hulled and sliced

¼ cup frozen raspberries

Juice of 1 navel orange

SERVES 4

If you are not crazy about salads, or about spinach in general, because you think it is boring and bland, try it with Hamilton, Ontario, native Margi Ende's dressing. You won't be sure if it is a salad or a fruit bowl.

Toss the spinach with the sliced strawberries in a serving bowl. Combine the raspberries and orange juice in a blender and puree until smooth. Toss with the spinach and the strawberries and serve.

TIP

Contrary to popular opinion, spinach is not a great source of iron. Although this leafy green supposedly kept Popeye the Sailor Man strong, spinach also contains oxalic acid, which binds with the iron in spinach and prevents the body from absorbing it. The only way to absorb calcium and iron from spinach is to eat it with vitamin C.

On the bright side, spinach has carotenoids, which help to keep eyes healthy. It also has loads of other vitamins and minerals that the body needs and can absorb.

MAC-
MACS

1 cup dried raw coconut flakes

1 cup raw macadamia nuts, chopped

½ cup almond flour

¼ cup raw agave nectar

1 tablespoon vanilla extract (see Tip, page 50)

1 tablespoon coconut oil

¼ teaspoon sea salt

MAKES 24 TO 30 COOKIES

Note that the nuts are not germinated in this recipe!

I have given you two types of "macs" to choose from. Some people love chocolate and some don't, believe it or not. I, for one, am not a chocolate person, but my friends are. I'd rather have them eat a raw healthy chocolate than a chocolate I know for sure is not good for them. So we have chocolate macs and fabulous nonchocolate Mac-Macs. Bravo, Christine. (She created both; I just love my sister.)

By the way, the toughest part of this recipe is walking away from the dehydrator for the 30 hours it takes to dehydrate the macaroons. You'll want to eat them before they're done. But restrain yourself; they are best when they finish their time in the dehydrator.

Mix the ingredients with your hands, or a spoon, in a large bowl. Form the mixture into 1-inch balls and place them on Teflex-lined dehydrator trays. Then flatten them with your hand or with a fork.

Dehydrate the cookies at 115 degrees F for approximately 12 hours or until at the desired gooeyness.

DEATH BY CHOCOLATE MACAROONS

2 cups dried raw coconut flakes

1 cup raw chocolate powder or raw carob powder

¾ cup raw agave nectar

1 tablespoon vanilla extract (see Tip, page 50)

2 tablespoons coconut oil

¼ teaspoon Himalayan salt

MAKES 24 COOKIES

The case for chocolate: It is said to be an aphrodisiac and anti-depressant. Cocoa butter in chocolate may prevent tooth decay by coating the teeth and preventing plaque from forming. And while cocoa butter has saturated fats, it also has phenolics, which may help lower the risk of heart disease.

I know Christine was thinking about all this when she created these delicious cookies!

Mix the coconut flakes, cocoa powder, agave nectar, vanilla, coconut oil, and salt in a large bowl with your hands or a spoon. Form the mixture into 1-inch balls and place them on Teflex-lined dehydrator trays. Flatten the cookies with your hand or with a fork and dehydrate at 115 degrees F for approximately 20 to 30 hours, depending on the size of the cookie.

16 PIZZA PERFECT LUNCH

RAW PIZZA

SERVES 8

1 cup golden flax seeds

1 cup purified water

2 cups raw almonds, germinated (see pages 41–43)

2 tablespoons chopped onion

2 tablespoons chopped fresh thyme

2 tablespoons chopped fresh rosemary

2 tablespoons chopped fresh oregano

Even though I am a raw foodist, I do cheat, but I try not to do it often. I like popcorn at hockey games, and once a year I treat myself to the best pizza I know and the one I grew up on—Borelli's Pizza on Hempstead Turnpike, right by the Nassau Coliseum on Long Island. Frank Borelli, the owner, has made me a fabulous rice-crust pizza, and now his other patrons with wheat allergies ask him to make it for them, too!

My point is if you're going to cheat, admit that you are cheating and keep it a once- or twice-a-week event. (And pop your enzymes; they will help you digest your cooked pizza.) The rest of the time, when you crave pizza, this will give you what you want. It has all the trappings of cooked pizza, but it won't burn the roof of your mouth!

Grind the flax seeds finely in a spice or coffee grinder. Soak the ground seeds in the water until it is completely absorbed, stirring occasionally; which should take about 2 hours. Place the soaked flax seeds in a food processor and add the almonds, onion, thyme, rosemary, and oregano. Process until the mixture is finely ground and well mixed.

TOPPINGS

Sun-Dried Tomato Sauce (recipe follows)

White Topping with Optional Fresh Tomatoes (recipe follows)

Dried oregano (optional)

Simple Olive Tapenade (recipe follows, optional)

Roll the dough in your hands to form 8 balls of equal size (it may help to wash your hands after rolling a few). Once all the balls are rolled, flatten them evenly with the palm of your hand.

Place the pizza breads on a Teflex-lined dehydrator tray and dehydrate them at 115 degrees F for about 4 hours. Then flip the breads over onto the dehydrator trays and remove the Teflex liners. Continue to dehydrate for another 4 hours, or until done. You can make bigger pizza breads, which will take longer to dehydrate.

Spread the Sun-Dried Tomato Sauce over the pizzas. Add the white topping and, if desired, top it with the finely chopped fresh tomato, a drizzle of olive oil, a dash of dried oregano, and olive tapenade.

sun-dried tomato sauce

1 cup sun-dried tomatoes

Put the sun-dried tomatoes in a bowl, barely cover them with purified water, and let them soak for at least 1 hour. Pour off half the water and put the tomatoes and the remaining water in a food processor. Blend the mixture until the tomatoes are chopped into a coarse paste.

white topping with optional fresh tomatoes

1 cup raw macadamia nuts

1 cup raw pine nuts

2 tablespoons nutritional yeast (optional)

1 tablespoon cold-pressed, extra-virgin olive oil

2 tablespoons fresh lemon juice

1 small garlic clove, minced

1 tablespoon Nama Shoyu

½ cup purified water

3 to 4 ripe plum tomatoes, finely chopped

Cover and soak the raw macadamia nuts and pine nuts in water for 1 hour. Drain the nuts and place them in a food processor with the yeast (if using), olive oil, lemon juice, garlic, Nama Shoyu, and water, blending them together until they are the consistency of ricotta cheese.

simple olive tapenade

After olive oil, olives are the next best thing. Believe me, most of the olives you get in the store are cooked, even if they don't look like it. At Carolalt.com you can get your hands on deliciously fabulous raw olives that are not flash-cooked in the jar. They are cured in brine and in my view, are much healthier for you.

This tapenade made with raw olives is a healthy snack that gives you your daily allotment of essential fatty acids. They are the building blocks of many things in your body, including your immune system. Don't kid yourself; you're surviving on cooked oils only because your body is extraordinarily efficient, not because you are giving your body what it needs!

2 cups raw pitted olives (black or green)

1 tablespoon Bragg Liquid Aminos (optional)

2 tablespoons cold-pressed, extra-virgin olive oil

Put the olives, and the Bragg Liquid Aminos if you are using it, in the blender and chop finely. Drizzle in the oil with the blender running until a think paste forms. Store the tapenade in a VacSy System container until needed. Tapenade will keep this way for 3 to 4 days.

TIPS

I love a strong-flavored olive like Moroccan or Greek for this recipe.

Tapenade is also great on crackers or bread.

WATERCRESS AND RED PEPPER SALAD

SERVES 4 TO 6

1 to 2 garlic cloves, pressed through a garlic press

1 small piece of gingerroot, pressed through a garlic press

Juice of ½ lemon

1 tablespoon flax seed oil

Nama Shoyu to taste (optional)

2 bunches watercress, coarsely chopped

3 medium red bell peppers, seeded and chopped

3 to 4 tablespoons very finely chopped onion

In a small bowl, thoroughly mix together the garlic, ginger, lemon juice, and flax seed oil, adding Nama Shoyu if desired. Set the dressing aside.

Toss the watercress, red peppers, and onion in a serving bowl. Drizzle the dressing over the salad and serve.

MASON'S BLUEBERRY BANANA SMOOTHIE

1 frozen banana

½ fresh ripe banana

Handful of fresh blueberries

TIP

Blueberries are just about as healthy as a food can be. Blueberries rank first in antioxidant activity when compared to forty other fresh fruits and vegetables. Antioxidants help neutralize harmful by-products of metabolism called free radicals, which can lead to cancer and a variety of age-related diseases.

SERVES 1

Eating raw is contagious. Once my coauthor David started, his family and all his friends tried it, too, and they each began creating recipes, including this really simple one from his stepson, Mason Mahaffey. This versatile smoothie can be served as a snack, a drink, or a dessert. The combination of frozen and fresh ripe bananas is what makes it so creamy. It will remind you of an old-fashioned shake right from the ice cream parlor. Best of all, it's so easy, even a kid could make it. (Wait, in fact, Mason is a kid!) You'll feel like one too when you slurp this smoothie down.

Combine the frozen and fresh bananas and blueberries in a blender and puree. Add as much purified water as needed (up to ½ cup) to achieve the thickness you prefer and blend again. When the liquid is smooth and frothy, pour the smoothie into a glass and serve.

17 LITE-N-EASY LUNCH

TUNA CEVICHE

1 cup fresh lemon juice (4 to 6 lemons)

1 cup fresh lime juice (6 to 8 limes)

1 garlic clove

1 jalapeño pepper, chopped

½ teaspoon Himalayan salt

1 pound boneless, skinless, sashimi-grade tuna

Kernels from 2 ears of corn

4 plum tomatoes, chopped

2 ripe avocados, pitted, peeled, and cubed

Chopped fresh cilantro for garnish (optional)

SERVES 6

I am not vegan, nor do I want to be fully vegan. I like fish protein, and I feel useless and tired without it. I also love the fish oils and prefer to get my oils from the natural source that God created, rather than from a man-made or man-processed source. I love it when people ask me what I eat, and I can say raw fish (sashimi, tartare, ceviche, marinated, lightly seared, and cured) and meat (carpaccio, bresaola, tartare, and seared) and dairy (raw milks, creams, butters, and raw-milk cheeses). Most of these are sold right in your grocery store—not hidden, just undiscovered!

Combine the lemon juice, lime juice, garlic, jalapeño, and salt in a blender, and pulse to mix them well. Cut the tuna into ½-inch cubes (the smaller the pieces of tuna, the faster they will "cook") and place in an airtight container with a tight-fitting lid. Cover the tuna with the juice mixture, making sure that all the tuna is fully immersed, and cover the container. Marinate until the tuna is "cooked" to your liking. Drain the tuna, reserving half of the lemon-lime mixture.

TIP

The easiest way to remove the pit from the avocado is to cut the avocado in half, hold the half with the pit in the palm of your hand, take an ordinary dinner knife (not the sharpest knife you have, so you don't cut yourself) and with blade side down, "chop" into the pit. When the knife is stuck in the pit, gently turn the knife clockwise, which will loosen the pit so that it comes out easily.

Toss the marinated tuna with the corn, tomatoes, and avocados in a large serving bowl. Top it with the reserved marinade, sprinkle it with cilantro to taste, if desired, and let everyone help themselves. Or you can serve individual portions in martini glasses or on plates on a bed of greens.

CUCUMBER AVOCADO SOUP

SERVES 4

This soup is so light and fresh that one thing you won't feel after eating it is "fat." But it has the kind of fat your body really needs.

Dr. Robert Marshall, whom I quoted in my first book, basically said that raw fats can cause a preferential exchange with unusable fats stuck in the body. That means that raw fats help the body to get rid of the bad, indigestable, stored fats by exchanging them for raw fats that can be used by the body as ready-made energy. As you use this fat for energy and rebuilding your body, you can become slimmer! In fact, the cooked fats were stored because they were useless to the body.

4 large cucumbers, cleaned and peeled

4 celery stalks

1 Hass avocado, peeled and pitted

¼ cup chopped dill

¼ cup fresh-squeezed lemon juice

4 cups purified water

Put all the ingredients in the blender and whir them until creamy smooth. Pour into bowls and serve.

TIP

The phrase "cool as a cucumber" refers to the fact that cucumbers have such a high water content they can remain 20 degrees cooler than the outside air when the temperature spikes. The cuke is a diminutive cousin to the watermelon, works as a diuretic, and has other cleansing properties. Besides being one of the most refreshing things to eat, it can be used topically to soothe burns and sores and soften the skin.

ROSEMARY CRACKERS

2 cups golden flax seeds

3 cups purified water

2 cups raw almonds, germinated (see pages 41–43)

1 teaspoon Himalayan salt

¼ cup fresh rosemary, coarsely chopped

MAKES 24

My sister Christine knows I like crackers and breads. Maybe that's why she makes so many different kinds. I love 'em, and because I like variety and abundance, I will keep searching out new and different recipes for crackers.

Again, because they are made from germinated almonds, these do count toward your daily dose of ten germinated almonds. These crackers are good alone or with hummus, tapenade, guacamole, or raw-milk cheeses. Enjoy!

Put the flax seeds in a spice or coffee grinder and finely grind them. Soak the ground flax seeds in the water for 1 hour or until all the water is absorbed. Drain the almonds and grind in a food processor with the soaked flax seeds, salt, and fresh rosemary until well mixed and finely chopped.

Spread the cracker mixture on Teflex-lined dehydrator trays as evenly and thinly as you can without leaving any holes. Dehydrate the cracker sheets at 115 degrees F for approximately 6 to 8 hours, or until the tops are dry to the touch. Flip the crackers onto the dehydrator trays and peel off the Teflex liners. Place the cracker sheets back in the dehydrator for approximately 3 to 4 more hours, or until the tops are a bit drier. Cut the sheets into small cracker-sized squares. Return the crackers to the dehydrator until they are crispy and crunchy, for approximately 6 to 10 hours.

PECAN PIE

2 cups raw almonds, germinated (see pages 41–43)

35 pitted dates, soaked for 1 hour and drained

1 tablespoon fresh lime juice

½ teaspoon ground cinnamon

¼ teaspoon Himalayan salt

½ teaspoon vanilla extract

2 cups raw pecans, germinated (see pages 41–43)

Cold-pressed extra-virgin olive oil to grease your pan

MAKES 20 TO 24 SQUARES

Still think that I suffer and do without? That I am deprived? That's how I feel about cooked-food eaters who deprive themselves by dieting. Those poor people suffering and doing without great deserts because they are fattening and unhealthy, while I am eating a raw Pecan Pie like this.

Eat your heart out, baby!

Combine the almonds and 10 of the dates in a food processor and process until they are coarsely ground and clumping together. Grease the bottom of a 9-inch square brownie pan or a pie plate with a little cold-pressed olive oil to keep the pie from sticking to the plate. Press the almond-and-date mixture evenly into the bottom of brownie pan and up the sides to form a crust. Set aside.

Combine the remaining dates, the fresh lime juice, cinnamon, salt, and vanilla in a blender or small food processor, and process until the mixture has a smooth, uniform consistency. Spread the date filling evenly over the crust. Arrange the raw pecans on top of the date mixture and press lightly. Cut the pie into 2-inch squares and serve.

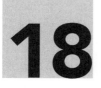18 THE IDEAL MEAL

2 large handfuls of lettuce and/or a baby greens mixture

Large handful of sunflower seeds, sprouted (see pages 41–43)

⅓ scallion (white and green parts), thinly sliced

⅓ medium cucumber, quartered and sliced

½ ripe avocado, pitted, peeled, and diced

2 to 3 tablespoons raw sauerkraut

¼ cup dulse, snipped into small pieces

5 to 7 raw pitted black olives

Drizzle of any high-quality, cold-pressed oil (optional)

TIPS

If you have never tasted raw sauerkraut, you must. It's available in the jar at health-food stores and at Whole Foods.

Dulse is a nutrient-dense red seaweed with a fine, light, briny sea taste. It is delicious on salads and soups, and may be eaten with cheese.

KELLY'S SALAD FOR ONE

SERVES 1

Because the stereotype of the raw foodist is someone who only eats salads, I hesitated to include a main-course salad among The Raw 50. *Let's face it, though, there are times when that's exactly what we want. And since this salad comes from master chef and author Kelly Serbonich, formerly of the Hippocrates Health Institute of Palm Beach, it's not just simple, it's simply a masterpiece. Enjoy!*

In a large bowl, toss all the ingredients together, except the oil. Drizzle with the oil if desired, and serve with Super Flax Crax.

KELLY'S SUPER FLAX CRAX

MAKES **8** TO **12** LARGE CRACKERS

These 'crax' speak for themselves. Read about the power of flax on page 37.

1 pound flax seeds, soaked for 4 to 6 hours and drained

¼ pound pumpkin seeds, soaked for 4 to 6 hours and drained

¼ pound raw pistachios, soaked for 4 to 6 hours and drained

¼ cup fresh lemon juice

1 red bell pepper, seeded and roughly chopped

¾ medium red onion, roughly chopped

1 garlic clove, minced

2 tablespoons ground cumin

¼ cup dulse flakes

¼ cup Bragg Liquid Aminos or Nama Shoyu

2½ cups purified water

½ bunch fresh parsley, stemmed and chopped

Grind the flax seeds in a spice grinder, coffee grinder, or blender. Transfer to a large bowl and set aside. In a food processor, combine the pumpkin seeds, pistachios, lemon juice, bell pepper, onion, garlic, cumin, dulse flakes, and Bragg Aminos or Nama Shoyu. Process until thoroughly combined, and add to the bowl of ground flax seeds. Add the water to the mixture, and then stir in the parsley. Let stand for at least 30 minutes. The batter should be thick and spreadable. If necessary, add a small amount of water to increase spreadability.

Spread out the batter on Teflex-lined dehydrator trays about ⅛ inch thick and dehydrate overnight. Flip over the crackers, peel off the Teflex sheets, and return the crackers to the dehydrator until fully dry and crispy another 2 to 3 hours. Break them up into pieces and store in an airtight container.

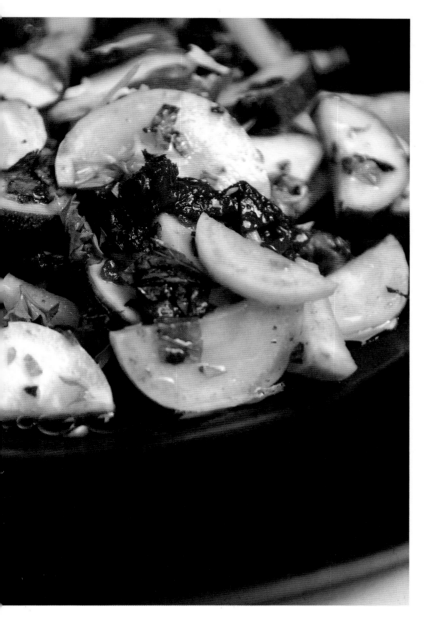

SPICED
SQUASH
PAGE 140

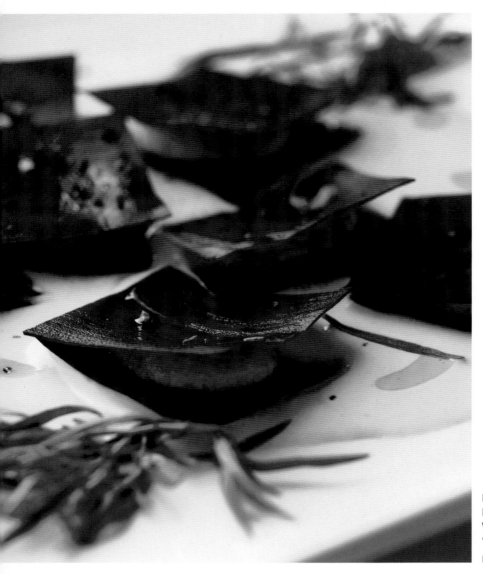

**RED BEET
RAVIOLI
WITH TARRAGON
"GOAT CHEESE"**

PAGE 110

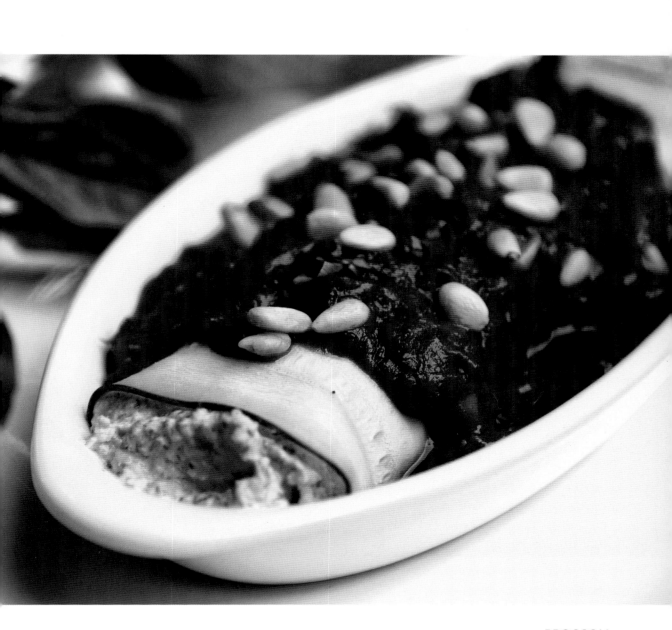

**BROCCOLI
CHEDDAR
CANNELLONI**

PAGE 138

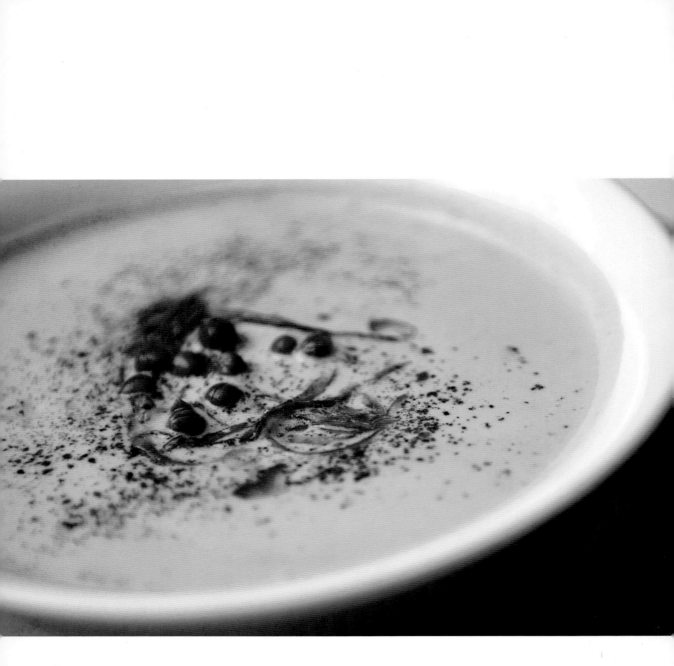

**CUCUMBER
AVOCADO SOUP**

PAGE 92

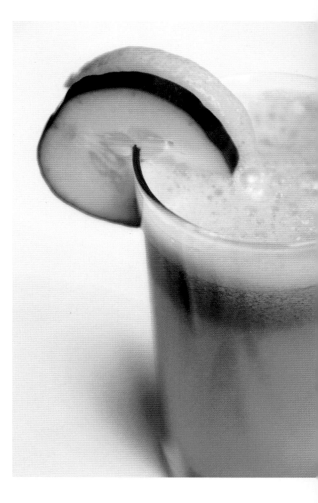

FOUNTAIN
OF YOUTH
SWEET
CUCUMBER
SUMMER JUICE

PAGE 157

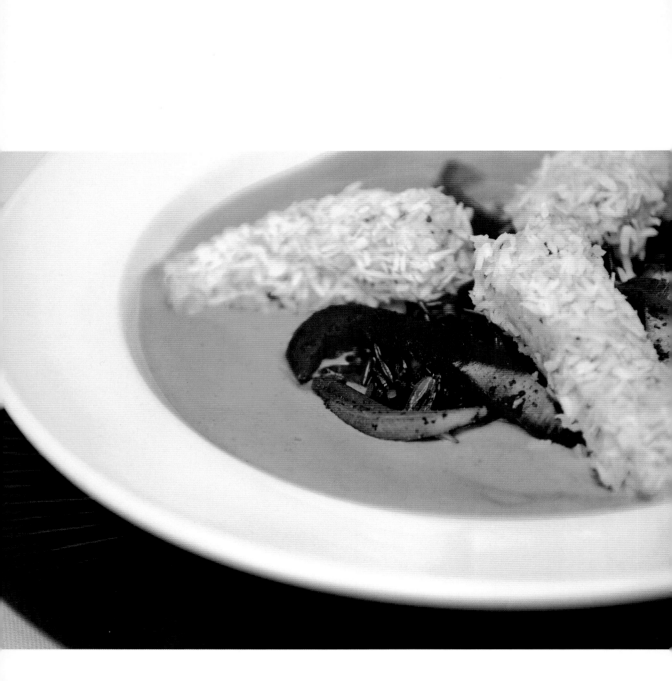

**COCONUT-CRUSTED "SHRIMP"
WITH RED CURRY SAUCE**

PAGE 119

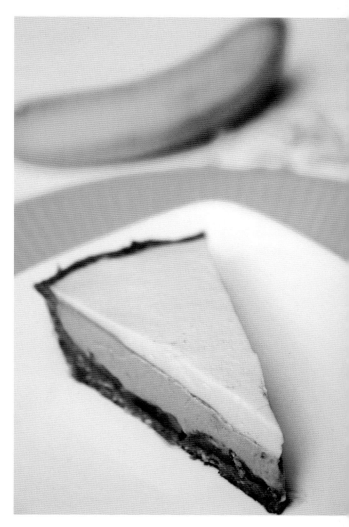

**"EASY AS PIE"
COOL LEMON
CREAM PIE**

PAGE 117

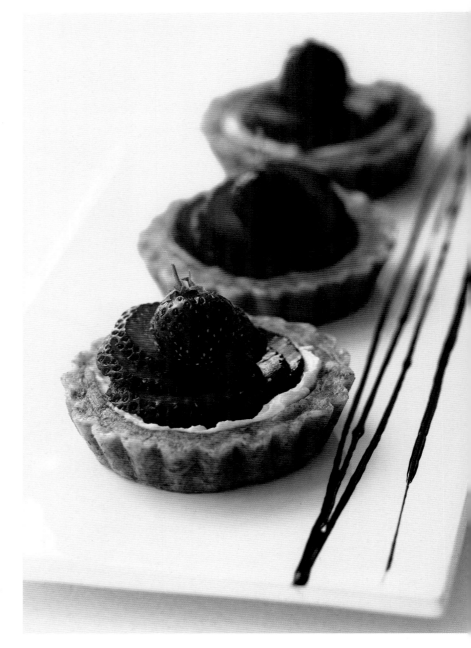

SARMA'S
STRAWBERRY
TARTS

PAGE 113

VITO'S AMAZING BROWNIES

2 cups shredded dried coconut

2 pitted Medjool dates

3 tablespoons raw liquid honey

1 tablespoon carob powder

1 teaspoon vanilla extract

TIP

To open a young coconut: On the flat end of the coconut, make a 5-point star cut into the outer husk, then use the pronged end of a hammer to rip off the husk a piece at a time. Once you are down to the inner brown shell, use the hammer and screwdriver to pierce one of the hard "eyes." Next, poke the screwdriver into the soft eye, being careful not to spill the liquid inside. Pour the liquid into a glass, then locate the two spines running lengthwise down the shell and use the hammer to crack the coconut in the prone area where there is no spine. Use a spoon to pry the off the broken shell pieces.

SERVES 8

I worked in a bakery when I was a teenager. And if I had snacked on Vito Natale's brownies, I would not have put on those extra twenty pounds, which I had to get rid of when I started modeling!

Many people ask me how it is possible to have a raw brownie. They wonder if I am talking about eating the batter. (Hate to ruin your day, but even common brownie batter is not raw, because some of the ingredients you use—like oil or butter—are already cooked before you get them.) Dehydrating does what baking does: dries out the batter so that it holds together and you can eat a brownie without it oozing through your fingers.

The difference between oven cooking and dehydrating is that dehydrating at low temperatures doesn't alter the pH (acidity or alkalinity) of the food. Nor does it kill enzymes or denature the vitamins and minerals in the food. The trade-off is that it takes longer to prepare. But, hey, aren't you worth it?

And after a salad, what's better than a guilt-free brownie?

Blend all the ingredients thoroughly in a blender or food processor until finely chopped and well combined. With your hands, form the mixture into 2 × 4-inch rectangles, each about ¾ inch thick. If they don't hold together, add a bit more honey to the mixture.

Place the brownies on Teflex-lined dehydrator trays and dehydrate at 105 degrees F for 6 to 8 hours, depending on how moist you like them.

A HIPPIE PICNIC

THYME BREAD

1 cup dark flax seeds

1 cup purified water

1 cup raw walnuts, germinated (see pages 41–43)

¼ cup fresh chopped thyme

1½ teaspoons Himalayan salt

SUNFLOWER PÂTÉ

1 cup sunflower seeds

3 large carrots

¼ cup fresh lemon juice

⅛ cup Bragg Liquid Aminos

¼ cup raw sesame tahini

¼ cup chopped scallions (white and green parts)

2 red onion slices

3 tablespoons chopped fresh parsley

1 to 2 garlic cloves, minced

¼ teaspoon cayenne pepper

Avocado slices

Tomato slices

Sprouts

Lettuce

THE SIMPLE VEGGIE SANDWICH

SERVES 4

I was once told that I could make a sandwich out of anything, and I can, because I love sandwiches. I know I'm not alone. Here's one you're sure to love. It's made on fresh, raw Thyme Bread and is another of my sister Christine's creations.

Put the flax seeds in spice or coffee grinder and grind finely. Soak the ground flax seeds in the water for 1 hour; all the water should be absorbed. Combine the soaked flax seeds, walnuts, thyme, and salt in a food processor and process until finely chopped and well mixed.

Spread the mixture thinly on Teflex-lined dehydrator trays and dehydrate at 115 degrees F for approximately 6 hours, or until the tops are dry to the touch. Flip the breads over onto the dehydrator screens and peel off the Teflex liners. Continue to dehydrate on the screens for another 3 hours. Cut the bread into the desired shape and size. Place back into dehydrator for about another 6 hours. The bread should be pliable, and not crunchy. If you desire crispier bread, dehydrate longer.

In a pinch, you can use Food for Life's delicious Ezekiel 4:9 or Genesis 1:29 breads, which are made from sprouted grains and seeds. (They are the only breads that I have found made from only sprouted ingredients.) While they're not raw, they are about as good a bread as you can find in the health-food store or a good supermarket.

You can use this pâté like butter; it adds not only flavor, but creamy moistness as well. It also contributes the power of raw sunflower seeds; their oils are immune-building essential fatty acids! They provide energy as well. When sunflower seeds are mixed with raw tahini, which is sesame seed paste, the combination gives you several different oils. Good for you, in many more ways then one!

Spread leftovers on flax seed crackers. This tasty pâté will keep well in the refrigerator for about 2 weeks.

Put all the pâté ingredients in a food processor, and process until well blended. Refrigerate if not using at once.

To assemble your sandwiches, spread the bread with the pâté. Top 4 slices with avocado and tomato slices, your favorite sprouts, and lettuce and a second slice of thyme bread.

BEET AND APPLE SALAD

2 tablespoons raw honey

2 tablespoons raw apple cider vinegar

1 tablespoons cold-pressed, extra-virgin olive oil

1 tablespoon Udo's Choice oil blend, or cold-pressed olive oil, or some of both

Salt and pepper to taste

2 pounds beets

1 apple

1 to 2 teaspoons chopped fresh parsley

TIP

A word of caution from your dry cleaner. If you eat an apple and a juicy bite sprays your clothing, in about two weeks a brown spot will appear. This spot, caused by the pectin in the apple, is impossible to get out. True, the chemical used in the dry cleaning actually brings out the spot, but the real culprit is the invisible apple pectin that dried on your clothing. I've ruined more than one piece of clothing this way.

SERVES 6 TO 8

This side dish is so sweet that it almost makes a dessert redundant! KellyAnn Palazzolo, my chiropractor's assistant, has created this original recipe. It calls for only olive oil, but I always mix oils—raw olive oil and Udo's Choice oil, because the latter is immune boosting. Udo's choice is a cold-pressed, seed-oil mixture. And when we talk about having a wide variety of oils and veggies, this is what I mean: Olive oil has some vitamins and minerals and essential fatty acids, but the body needs more. It needs all the diverse essential fatty acids and all the vitamins and minerals you can feed it.

Combine the honey, vinegar, and olive oil in a small bowl. Season with salt and pepper and set aside.

Peel and slice the beets thinly and put in a salad bowl. Peel and slice the apples thinly and add to the beets.

Toss the apples and beets with the dressing, sprinkle with the parsley, and serve.

20 THE RAW MEXICAN LUNCH

GUACAMOLE AND LETTUCE BURRITOS

3 small ripe avocados

1 ripe tomato

½ small jalapeño pepper, seeded and finely chopped

1½ teaspoons organic onion powder or diced onion

1 tablespoon fresh lemon juice

2 fresh cilantro sprigs, stemmed and finely chopped

¾ teaspoon Himalayan salt

6 romaine lettuce leaves

SERVES 6

No one can live without Mexican food, and the raw foodist is no exception! Raw foodists come in a variety of shapes, sizes, habits, and nationalities, and so does their food. These ingredients are the same as those in "normal" cooked Mexican food. We simply exchanged raw for cooked ingredients. Come see for yourself.

Halve the avocados and remove the pits. Use a spoon to scoop the flesh into a mixing bowl and mash lightly with a fork. Halve the tomato through the equator and cut the tomato halves into ½-inch dice. Add to the avocados and then add the jalapeño, onion powder, lemon juice, and salt. Combine the ingredients gently, mashing a bit more if you like your guacamole less chunky. Heap the guacamole onto the romaine leaves and wrap each leaf around the filling like a burrito.

EVERYDAY **CHILI**

1 small eggplant, peeled and cut into ¼-inch dice

5 fresh shiitake mushrooms, or 1 medium portabello mushroom, stemmed and cut into ¼-inch dice

1 medium zucchini, cut into ¼- to ½-inch pieces

3 garlic cloves, crushed

¼ medium red onion, finely chopped

1 medium plum tomato, cut into ¼- to ½-inch chunks

MARINADE

1 tablespoon fresh lemon juice

2 tablespoons cold-pressed, extra-virgin olive oil

3½ teaspoons Himalayan salt

SERVES 6

If you notice, this recipe differs from the first chili recipe in this section (see Sweet Melissa's Autumn Chi-lee on page 62), yet they are both a version of the popular cooked chili. Just as cooked food has diverse recipes for the same thing, so does raw food. Actually, that is the only way that I can think of that raw and cooked foods are alike!

You need to try things and decide for yourself what you like because you will not like everything. I can't imagine you like every piece of cooked food set down in front of you, and raw food is no different. I repeat, you need to try things to find what you like!

Combine the eggplant, mushrooms, zucchini, garlic, onion, and tomato in a quart-sized jar or container with a cover.

For the marina, whisk the lemon juice, olive oil, and Himalayan salt in a small bowl, and pour it over the vegetables. Cover and marinade at room temperature for at least 6 hours and preferably overnight.

SAUCE

1 large tomato, cut in chunks

1 cup sun-dried tomatoes, soaked in purified water for 20 minutes, and drained

¼ cup cold-pressed, extra-virgin olive oil

⅛ to ¼ teaspoon cayenne pepper

1 teaspoon fresh oregano leaves

1½ teaspoon chili powder

Cashew Sour Cream (recipe follows) for serving (optional)

Just before serving, make the sauce: Put the fresh and sun-dried tomatoes in the bowl of a food processor and process until finely chopped. Add the olive oil, cayenne pepper, oregano, and chili powder and whir to make a puree. Pour the pureed sauce over the marinated vegetables and stir to combine; discard the garlic cloves.

Transfer the chili to a saucepan and warm to no more than 115 degrees F, using a deep-fat thermometer. (You can also heat the chili in a temperature-controlled Crock-Pot.) Taste for seasoning, adding more salt or cayenne if needed. Spoon into bowls and top each serving with a dollop of Cashew Sour Cream, if desired.

cashew sour cream

The great thing about cashews is their versatility. You can make a sour cream for a soup or chili or a whipped cream for dessert just by changing the other ingredients you mix with it. But be careful, too much of anything is not so good. Cashews are very fatty and that is good, but too much of one type of fat is not good for you. Variety, variety!

1 cup raw cashews

⅓ cup fresh coconut meat, preferably from a young Thai coconut

½ teaspoon raw apple cider vinegar

½ teaspoon unpasteurized light miso paste

¼ teaspoon Himalayan salt

Juice of ½ lemon

Soak the cashews in purified water for a minimum of 2 hours and as long as overnight. The water should cover the nuts by ½ inch. Drain any leftover water from the cashews, then place the nuts in the blender with the remaining ingredients. Whirl until they come together in a smooth and creamy puree. Keep in the fridge in a VacSy container or eat it up while it is fresh.

RASPBERRY SORBET

MAKES 6 SMALL SERVINGS

1½ cups organic raspberries, plus 6 for garnish

1½ tablespoons raw liquid honey

⅓ cup purified water at room temperature

The first time I made this recipe, I was skeptical about it. Would it taste like the sorbet I grew up on? Would it be as fabulous as the sorbet I remembered but have not eaten for years because it is full of sugar, is fattening, and bad for my hypoglycemia?

Well, no it wasn't the same; it was better! It had more real-fruit taste and it was creamier. And the best part was that it was something I had made myself, and I didn't mess it up with any additives! I took a lot of satisfaction in that.

Freeze the raspberries (except those for garnish) overnight. When they're ready, stir the honey into the water until it is dissolved. Combine the frozen raspberries and honey water in a blender and whir until the berries and liquid have a smooth, sherbetlike consistency. Add a little more water if needed, being careful not to let the sorbet become too soft. Divide among 6 dishes, and garnish each scoop with a fresh berry on top. Serve right away!

TIP

Sometimes I buy organic frozen berries at Whole Foods and blend them. Make sure you get the kind that do not have any added syrup or sugar!

PENNI SHELTON IRRITABLE BOWEL SYNDROME
Tulsa, Oklahoma

Penni's health problems started early.

By age eight she suffered from persistent, unexplainable intestinal problems. "I would often miss the school bus because I was struggling with cramps, pain, and diarrhea," she says. "My stomach problems created tremendous stress for me on so many levels. The doctors performed lots of tests, but there was never a clear diagnosis."

Penni's symptoms continued throughout adolescence and into adulthood, especially when she ate or was under stress. Unable to identify the cause of her ailments, she spent many nights lying in bed, curled up in terrible pain, unable to do anything but pray. "My prayers usually consisted of nothing more than simple cries for relief," she recalls.

As the years passed she learned to manage her embarrassing problem. She learned not to accept invitations to any function where she would not have ready access to a bathroom. She made sure she drove her own car wherever she went. And out of fear that she might suffer another attack, she made certain not to eat anything when traveling. She lived with the constant fear that she would double over in pain or lose control of her bowels.

When she was in her early twenties, she learned that her problem was called irritable bowel syndrome (IBS) and it was treatable. But the medications she was prescribed over the years had side effects that were not much more appealing than the problem itself. Nor did they entirely alleviate her IBS symptoms; they merely helped to hold the IBS at bay. By the time she reached her late thirties, with a life that most people would find enviable, Penni felt she was spiraling out of control.

"I was reflecting upon all that God had blessed me with: a beautiful, healthy daughter, a wonderful marriage, a thriving professional life, and a deep, rich faith. At the same time, though, I found myself at the unhealthiest point in my life. My IBS was relentless and debilitating, my weight was soaring to new levels, and my use of alcohol to numb my symptoms had become a daily crutch." she recalls. "I was in a depression and felt a real sense of hopelessness for the first time in my life. I was doing a good job of putting on a game face each morning, but inside I felt like things were falling apart."

While preparing for a family vacation in August, Penni stopped by the local bookstore to pick up a few magazines for the trip, and a book caught her eye. "It had Carol Alt on the cover, Penni says. "As a teenager I had Carol Alt posters plastered on my bedroom walls, so just out of curiosity, I picked up a copy along with my magazines."

Later, settled on a lounge chair in the sun, Penni opened *Eating in the Raw* and began reading. What she learned changed her life.

"I kept reading parts of it aloud to my husband as the children played in the water park. I could tell he found it as intriguing as I did. The words seemed to penetrate not only my mind but my heart as well. I asked myself, Could the lack of healthy, raw, alive, enzyme-rich foods have been the source of my problems for all these years? I began to look at my surroundings with a new eye. All around me gigantic, unhealthy parents and children jiggled between the funnel cake hut and the Dippin' Dots kiosk. I counted five men who clearly had fairly recent open-heart surgeries, all overweight, noshing on junk food. 'Oh my God,' I thought, 'I'm surrounded by sick food, sick people, and I am sitting right here in the middle of hell,' " Penni says.

Penni and husband, Gordon, decided then and there to start eating raw, knowing that they had nothing to lose. "I felt as though I had tried everything else," she recalls, "so I might as well take Carol's advice and eat in a way that might enable me to live my life fully alive and not just eat to survive."

The Sheltons immediately began eating almost completely raw. Within the first week, all of Penni's lifelong irritable bowel syndrome symptoms were gone. Within eight weeks she lost fifteen unwanted pounds, and she had not reduced the amount of food she was eating at all. In fact, she finally felt free to eat and enjoy food as she never had before. "We ate and ate wonderfully healthy, raw foods, as much as we wanted, and the weight was still falling off," she recalls.

Penni had to relearn everything about preparing food for herself and her family. In their hometown of Tulsa, Oklahoma, there were no raw restaurants. "I knew it would be up to me to figure out how to make this work," she says, so she read everything she could find on raw food and she outfitted her kitchen. She learned how to shop all over again. She got into an entirely new groove of meal planning and food preparation. She tried recipes, and she began to create her own. Now she's as much at home with raw food as she was with cooked, and she feels one hundred times better.

"I still occasionally indulge in a cooked-food item here and there, but I choose wisely and I always take my enzymes when I know I'll be faced with eating something that isn't raw," she says.

Beautiful as she begins her forties, Penni Shelton doesn't look or feel her age. "I'm not hard-core about maintaining this lifestyle," she says. "I am a real person with a real life and what I have come to realize is that I really do like it raw."

10 RAW DINNERS

I eat a lot of dinners out. Wherever I do, I am always able to find something raw on the menu. In many of the cities I visit, I am always able to find some excellent places to eat, and I don't eat "like a model." **I eat, and I eat well. I do not hesitate to have dessert. I make sure I am always satisfied.** Because I'm eating raw food, though, I never feel full or bloated. I'm in the enviable position of having the best of both worlds. I don't have to eat like a pauper to look and feel great.

It's actually easy to eat dinner like a pauper. When I get to dinner, if I have done the right things all day, I am not so hungry. The problem for many people is they can't eat smaller amounts of food at night because they are simply too hungry. The combination of eating nonnutritious, cooked foods and skipping breakfast or lunch is the culprit. Eating well and correctly keeps your appetite in check and is a great weight-control device.

The Raw 50 dinner menus are shamelessly self-indulgent. Some of them come from the master chefs in my favorite restaurants. Every dish is so good that if you serve it to your cooked-food-eating friends, they probably won't believe you when you tell that that the food is raw. What an easy way to impress them! Some of the dishes are simpler to make than others. A few might be a challenge if you're new to preparing raw food, but every one of them is an exquisite example of how incredibly delicious entirely raw food can and should be.

Buon appetito.

A "PURE" DINING EXPERIENCE

RED BEET RAVIOLI WITH TARRAGON "GOAT CHEESE"

3 cups raw pine nuts

¾ cup cold-pressed, extra-virgin olive oil

2 whole lemons, zested, then peeled and quartered

1 medium shallot

2 tablespoons nutritional yeast

2 teaspoons whole black peppercorns

1 garlic clove

¾ cup purified water

Salt to taste

1 medium or 2 small red beets

¾ cup fresh tarragon leaves

Cracked pepper to taste

SERVES 6 TO 8

I was delighted when Sarma Melngailis, chef and cocreator of Pure Food and Wine as well as Chief Duck at oneluckyduck.com, gave me this recipe. The very thinly sliced vegetable that is used for the ravioli—in this case, red beet—has pretty much the same consistency as pasta. By the way, pasta means "paste" in Italian, and that's exactly what it is when it's in your system.

The real gift here is the "goat cheese," which is made with softened pine nuts. The last time I ate this dish, the "cheese" was so delicious, I ate it without the ravioli shell. Like cashews, pine nuts are extremely versatile, taking on the flavor of the spices you use with them. You can also mix them with mushrooms and make mushroom ravioli.

Soak the pine nuts in enough purified water to cover them for 1 hour. Drain, put the pine nuts in a food processor, and add the olive oil, lemon quarters, shallot, and zest. Process for about 8 minutes until the mixture is well combined and clumps together. Pour half of this mixture into a blender and set the rest aside. Add the yeast and 1 teaspoon of the

TIP

Compared to cooked or canned beets, raw beets have twice as much folic acid—a key vitamin in cellular development and repair—and potassium, which reduces anxiety, irritability, and stress and increases muscle strength.

peppercorns to the mixture in the blender and blend on medium speed for 2 minutes, until thick and smooth. Transfer the "goat cheese" to a bowl and refrigerate, uncovered, for 1 hour.

Meanwhile, place the reserved pine nut mixture in the blender. Add the remaining teaspoon of peppercorns, the garlic, and the water, and blend on high speed for 1 minute, until smooth but quite liquid. Add the salt, and set the sauce aside.

Roughly chop the tarragon and fold ½ cup of the leaves into the cheese once the cheese has completely chilled. Add salt to taste.

Peel the beets and slice paper-thin. Lay out half of the slices on a clean surface. Spoon about 1 tablespoon of the cheese onto each slice, then top each with a second beet slice. Arrange on a baking sheet in a single layer, sprinkle with salt, then store in the refrigerator.

To serve, pour the sauce onto a deep serving platter and arrange the ravioli on top. Sprinkle with the remaining ¼ cup of tarragon leaves, and salt and cracked pepper.

BABY SPINACH AND ARUGULA SALAD WITH CINNAMON BALSAMIC DRESSING AND CANDIED WALNUTS

SALAD

1 cup walnuts, soaked for 4 hours, drained, and dehydrated for 24 hours at 115 degrees F

2 tablespoons raw agave nectar

1 teaspoon ground cinnamon

1 teaspoon ground cardamom

¼ pound baby spinach

¼ pound baby arugula

1 small red onion, sliced paper-thin

1 Bosc pear, peeled, then shaved into ribbons with a vegetable peeler

DRESSING

½ cup cold-pressed, extra-virgin olive oil

2 tablespoons balsamic vinegar

1 tablespoon raw agave nectar

½ teaspoon ground cinnamon

¼ cup fresh tarragon leaves, roughly chopped

SERVES 4

I try to stay away from vinegar. It is acidic, and the body makes more than enough acid. But I understand that people like the taste and pucker that vinegar brings to a dish, so I've added this salad with balsamic vinegar because it really is delicious. Bear in mind that if you live a stressful life, the last thing you need is to be giving yourself additional acid. Perhaps you can substitute raw apple cider vinegar or lemon for the balsamic. At least they're raw.

If you don't have time to candy the walnuts, just toss them with agave and spices; they won't be caramelized and crunchy, but they will be sweet.

For the salad, toss the walnuts with the agave, cinnamon, and cardamom in a small bowl. Lay them on a Teflex-lined tray and dehydrate at 110 degrees F for 3 hours to caramelize. Set them aside. Gently toss the spinach, arugula, onion, and pear together, taking care not to bruise the spinach.

Whisk all the ingredients for the dressing together by hand or mix in a blender on low speed. Drizzle the dressing over the salad, and then top with the warm candied walnuts.

SARMA'S
STRAWBERRY TARTS

MAKES 12 TO 14 3-INCH TARTS

This is a true gourmet dessert, and you should have all the ingredients in your raw pantry except the strawberries. Make this in spring, when you can get fresh, local berries.

TART CRUST

4 cups whole raw almonds

¼ cup raw agave nectar

½ cup coconut oil at room temperature or slightly warmer

¼ teaspoon fine Himalayan salt

VANILLA CREAM

4 cups fresh coconut meat

½ cup light raw agave nectar

2 tablespoons vanilla extract

Seeds from ½ vanilla bean

½ teaspoon fine Himalayan salt

½ cup coconut oil, warmed until liquid

STRAWBERRIES

1 quart strawberries, hulled and sliced (1 large strawberry or 2 small ones for each tart)

¼ cup raw agave nectar

For the crust, grind the almonds in a food processor until fine, but stop before the they become too oily. (If you keep blending, it will become almond butter.) Transfer the ground nuts to a bowl and add the nectar, coconut oil, and salt.

Line about twelve 3-inch tart pans with plastic wrap, laying each sheet loosely over the tops, without tucking it under the pan. (If you don't have a tart pan, a muffin pan will do.) Fill each tart pan with 3 tablespoons of dough, and mold into the pan. Refrigerate for 30 minutes or until firm. Remove the crust from the pan by pulling up the plastic, then peel off plastic.

Combine all the vanilla cream ingredients except the coconut oil in a blender and puree until smooth. Add the coconut oil and blend until fully incorporated. Chill thoroughly for about 1 hour.

To assemble the tarts, fill each crust with 2 tablespoons of the vanilla cream. Top each tart with strawberry slices, overlapping them attractively. Drizzle with agave and refrigerate for 2 hours or until ready to serve.

TIP

You can freeze the tart shells for later use.

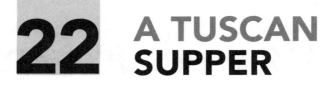

22 A TUSCAN SUPPER

PINE NUT "PARMIGIANO" (OPTIONAL)

1 cup raw pine nuts

SQUASH SPAGHETTI

1 medium butternut squash

½ cup cold-pressed, extra-virgin olive oil

4 garlic cloves, pressed through a garlic press

1 teaspoon Himalayan salt

TIPS

When people come to me with an ailment or complaint, I ask them if they eat wheat. Usually they say no right away. But then I ask, "No bread, crackers, cakes, cookies, canned soups or gravies, or pasta?" Then the lightbulb goes on—of course they eat wheat, it can be in all these foods, and also in items they may not suspect, like soy sauce.

The "parmigiano" can remain stored in the refrigerator for up to 1 month. Try to use a VacSy system to make sure they stay fresh!

SQUASH SPAGHETTI WITH GARLIC AND OIL AND PINE NUT "PARMIGIANO"

SERVES 4

When I cut wheat out of my diet, many of my health complaints disappeared, especially my sinus problems. What price did I pay for this freedom? Hardly anything! I gave up my daily pasta and substituted a raw pasta dish. The long, spaghetti-like veggies took on the flavor of whatever sauce I added. This dish looks and tastes a lot like pasta. You do need a spiral slicer; any kitchen store sells it, and it is easy to use. (You can also use it to make garnishes for your salads or other dishes.)

Don't be skeptical about the "parmigiano." It will change your mind not only about raw but also about how you eat nuts.

For the "parmigiano," soak the pine nuts in purified water for 8 hours. Rinse, drain, and germinate for 8 hours. Rinse again. Dehydrate in the dehydrator for 24 to 36 hours at 95 degrees F until thoroughly dry. Grind the nuts in a coffee grinder.

For the squash spaghetti, peel the squash and use a Saladaccio or similar spiral slicer to create spaghetti-like strands. In a large bowl, mix the olive oil, garlic, and salt. Toss in the squash spaghetti and mix until the strands are coated. Add the Pine Nut "Parmigiano" if you like.

JANICE INNELLA'S TUSCAN BREAD

3 cups golden flax seeds

½ cups pumpkin seeds

3 cups raw Brazil nuts, germinated for 24 hours, and then sprouted for 4 (see pages 41–43)

1 jalapeño pepper

1 tablespoon ground caraway seeds

1 bunch fresh basil, stemmed

1 bunch fresh rosemary, stemmed

½ cup sage leaves

1 cup cold-pressed olive oil

3 tablespoons Himalayan salt, or to taste

MAKES ABOUT 12 PIECES

Viva Italia! Nothing is tastier than Italian bread, and this one from Janice Innella of Essential Living Breads is delicious enough for any table in Siena. And with all these seeds and oils, this raw one is just so good for you. It helps build your immune system and is great for younger-looking skin. We know good skin is promoted when we protect it from the inside as well as the outside. You can leave some of the Brazil nuts ungerminated and chop them for a little crunch in your bread. Or add raw olives for a wonderful olive bread.

Soak 2 cups of the flax seeds in enough purified water to cover them for 4 hours, or until the water is completely absorbed. Combine the remaining cup of flax seeds with the pumpkin seeds in a spice or coffee grinder and whir until finely ground. (You may need to do this in batches.) Transfer to a large bowl. Grind the Brazil nuts and add to the bowl. Next, grind up the jalapeño, caraway seeds, and herbs, and add to the bowl. Add the soaked flax seeds, oil, and salt and mix by hand until you have a nice, uniform batter.

Spread out the batter evenly on Teflex-lined dehydrator trays as thick or thin as you like. Dry for 12 hours, then flip over the breads and peel off the Teflex sheets. Return to the dehydrator trays and dehydrate for another 12 hours, or until firm and bready but still moist.

FIELD GREENS SALAD WITH CREAMY BLACK PEPPER AND SAGE DRESSING

CREAMY BLACK PEPPER AND SAGE DRESSING

6 tablespoons raw sesame tahini

2 tablespoons light miso paste

About 24 fresh sage leaves

1 teaspoon Himalayan salt

2 tablespoons cold-pressed, extra-virgin olive oil

3 to 4 teaspoons freshly ground black pepper

Juice of 2 lemons

1½ tablespoons raw agave nectar

4 cups mixed mesclun salad greens

SERVES 4

Okay, you found my two favorite dressings: this one from Charlene Edgerton of Winston-Salem, North Carolina, and the Caesar Salad Dressing I wrote about in Eating in the Raw. *(There is a version of it on page 124.) You can tell from these dressings that I love creamy stuff. This dressing also makes an excellent pasta sauce.*

You simply cannot complain that raw recipes are too complicated. I won't hear it. What can be simpler than this?

Thank you, Charlene Edgerton, for sharing this recipe.

Combine the tahini, miso, and sage in a blender and whir until creamy. Add the salt, oil, pepper, lemon juice, and agave nectar and blend again, adding a bit of water if necessary; be careful not to make the dressing too runny.

Rinse and spin the greens, and transfer to a serving bowl. Toss with the dressing and serve.

TIP

You can buy a wide variety of fresh, organic greens at most good produce markets, and many vendors now sell them premixed. The advantage of buying the greens premixed is that you get a variety that is fresh, and you're less likely to have greens go bad in your fridge.

"EASY AS PIE" COOL LEMON CREAM PIE

Handful of raw almonds

Handful of pitted dates

2 tablespoons raw carob powder

1 ripe banana

½ cup shredded raw coconut meat

2 tablespoons fresh lemon juice

1 tablespoon flax seed oil

TIP

The banana packs a lot of energy: sucrose, fructose, and glucose, three natural sugars that not only get you going quickly but give you a boost that lasts. Athletes eat bananas because they provide an energy boost good enough for a ninety-minute workout.

SERVES 8

Dates are an amazing fruit, healthy and versatile. They become the paste that holds together the raw crusts for tarts and pies. Sometimes you'll find them in a cracker. They add just the right touch of sweetness, yet they're not overpowering. I was never a big fan of dates when I was growing up, but in the last few years I have radically changed my mind. (See tips on dates on page 174.)

Thank you Raw Chef Dan Hoyt for this and the next four recipes.

Combine the cashews, almonds, dates, and carob powder in the food processor and finely chop until the mixture is crumblike. Add purified water by the teaspoon until the mixture sticks together. Dump the crumbs into a glass pie plate and press onto the bottom and up the sides to form a crust.

Place the crust in the freezer for 5 to 10 minutes.

While the crust chills, combine the banana, coconut, lemon juice, and flax seed oil in a blender and whir until the texture is smooth and creamy. Fill the pie shell with the mixture, then refrigerate for 30 minutes or longer. Serve cold, cut into wedges.

23 QUINTESSENTIAL MEAL

1 medium tomato, coarsely chopped

1 bunch arugula, stems removed

1 red bell pepper, seeded and cut into chunks

2 medium cucumbers, cut into chunks

2 celery stalks, cut into chunks

¼ cup fresh lemon juice

¼ cup cold-pressed, extra-virgin olive oil

1 teaspoon salt

½ small tomato, cut in small dice for garnish

Cayenne pepper for garnish

Sprouted Kamut Flatbreads (page 67)

ARUGULA VEGGIE SOUP

SERVES 2

Jack LaLanne says eat five raw servings of fruits and veggies every day, and here they are, in all their glory.

Set aside 1 tablespoon of the chopped tomato for garnish. Combine the arugula, the remaining chopped tomato, the bell pepper, cucumbers, celery, lemon juice, and oil in a blender. Puree until finely chopped and well combined.

Divide the soup between two soup bowls and serve topped with some diced tomato and a dash of cayenne, with the flatbreads on the side.

TIP

Made from ground chile pods, cayenne pepper boosts circulation and blood flow, thus helping other herbs and supplements work more effectively. It has been used to treat toothaches, headaches, sore throats, and chronic pain.

COCONUT-CRUSTED "SHRIMP" WITH RED CURRY SAUCE

"SHRIMP"

1 cup sunflower seeds, germinated (see pages 41–43)

1 cup Brazil nuts, germinated (see pages 41–43)

Meat of 1 fresh young Thai coconut

¼ cup dulse

1 tablespoon red onion, coarsely chopped

¼ teaspoon peeled and chopped fresh gingerroot

1 medium garlic clove

1 cup dried raw coconut flakes

CURRY SAUCE

1 cup coconut water

¼ cup dried raw coconut flakes

1 red bell pepper, including seeds, cut into chunks

1 tablespoon cold-pressed, extra-virgin olive oil

1 tablespoon chopped red onion

2 tablespoons curry powder

1 teaspoon coconut butter

1 teaspoon Himalayan salt

1 teaspoon paprika

SERVES 2

Raw Chef Dan Hoyt made this one day in front of a classroom full of people. It was quick and easy to make and tasted delicious. Once everyone in the room had "ummmed" and "ahhhhhed" their way through the dish, I was prompted to ask Dan for this recipe for my book.

I eat most fish except scavenger fish like crustaceans. In other words, I eat fish with fins and scales. To me they're cleaner because the water flows through them. Crustaceans are stuck on the ground eating everything that falls to the bottom. And I do mean everything. I guess one fish's garbage is another fish's food, so I prefer the more picky fish. If we are what we eat, then so are they.

For the shrimp, combine the sunflower seeds, Brazil nuts, coconut meat, dulse, onion, ginger, and garlic in a blender or food processor. Shape into "shrimp" and roll in the coconut flakes. Place on Teflex-lined dehydrator trays and dehydrate at 95 degrees F for 12 hours.

When almost ready to serve, combine all the curry sauce ingredients in the blender and whir until smooth and creamy. Pour some curry sauce on each plate and top with "shrimp." Serve additional sauce at the table.

"SAUTÉED" VEGGIES

2 small heads
bok choy, sliced

1 red bell pepper, seeded
and sliced

1 yellow bell pepper, seeded
and sliced

1 yellow summer squash,
halved and sliced lengthwise
into half-moons

3 scallions (white and green
parts), cut on the diagonal
into 2-inch lengths

2 tablespoons cold-pressed,
extra-virgin olive oil

Himalayan salt and
freshly ground black
pepper to taste

SERVES 4

This is just the right side dish for the "shrimp" on page 119. The most time-consuming part of making this recipe is dehydrating the veggies. I think Raw Chef Dan Hoyt prepares these the night before, but that's okay, just put them in the dehydrator and go watch your movie!

Combine the vegetables in a bowl and drizzle with the oil. Toss to coat the vegetables, sprinkle with salt and pepper, and toss again.

Spread the vegetables on Teflex sheet dehydrator trays and dehydrate at 95 degrees F for 1 to 2 hours.

TIP

If green peppers "repeat" on you or make you burp, it is because green peppers are not fully ripe. Yellow, orange, red, and purple peppers have more enzymes, so they are sweeter and easier to digest.

RAW CHEF DAN'S ALMOND COCONUT COOKIES

1 cup raw almonds

½ cup dried raw coconut flakes

3 pitted dates

1½ teaspoons Himalayan salt

2 teaspoons vanilla extract

MAKES 8 COOKIES

When your cookies are made from nutritious raw foods they are not "fattening" in the same way that cooked cookies are. These almond cookies nourish your body—and taste great.

Combine all the ingredients in a food processor and process until well mixed and doughlike. Form into 1-inch-thick balls and flatten into cookies, place on Teflex-lined dehydrator trays, and dehydrate at 95 degrees F for 15 to 18 hours.

Variation: For softer cookies, first process the nuts and coconut flakes in a food processor to make a dry powder, then add the salt, vanilla, and 1 teaspoon of raw agave nectar or honey. Omit the dates. Mix with a fork, then shape and dehydrate as above.

24 ITALIAN-STYLE DINNER

HEATHY'S RAW LASAGNA

MUSHROOM LAYER

1 cup button mushrooms, thinly sliced

¼ cup Bragg Liquid Aminos

¼ cup chopped pitted kalamata olives

SAUCE

2 cups sun-dried tomatoes, soaked for 1 hour and drained

½ to ¾ cup chopped fresh tomatoes

2 pitted dates

½ cup fresh basil leaves, chopped

¼ cup pitted kalamata olives

1 to 2 garlic cloves, chopped

Himalayan salt to taste

Heather Pace is from Ontario, Canada, close to where I live. Too bad I didn't know that, as I love lasagna and couldn't find anyone who served a raw version. Now I use this recipe to satisfy my lasagna urges. This recipe needs to be shared with the world! It fulfills a civil service!

For the mushroom layer, mix the mushrooms and Bragg Liquid Aminos together in a medium bowl, and marinate for approximately 1 hour in the fridge.

Meanwhile, for the sauce, combine the ingredients in a food processor, adding just ½ cup of the fresh tomatoes to start. Process until finely chopped and saucelike, adding as much of the remaining tomatoes as needed to achieve the right consistency. The sauce should be thick to prevent the liquid from seeping out of the finished lasagna.

To make the ricotta, blend the nuts and lemon juice with just enough water to create a creamy paste with the consistency of thick ricotta cheese. Add enough salt to get that salty cheesy taste. Fold in the spinach.

For the noodles, use a mandoline to slice the eggplant and the zucchini lengthwise to make thin sheets. Reserve separately.

NUT RICOTTA

1½ cups cashews, soaked 4 to 8 hours and drained

½ cup walnuts, soaked 4 to 8 hours and drained

¼ cup fresh lemon juice

¼ to ½ cup purified water

Himalayan salt to taste

⅓ cup finely chopped spinach

NOODLES

1 eggplant, peeled

1 large zucchini, peeled

TOPPING

¼ cup chopped pitted kalamata olives

½ cup grated zucchini

To assemble the lasagna, spread a few tablespoons of the tomato sauce on the bottom of a 9 × 13-inch baking pan. Arrange a layer of eggplant noodles to cover the entire bottom of the pan. Top with a layer of tomato sauce.

Stir the ¼ cup of chopped olives into the mushroom mixture and spread evenly in the pan. Top with half the zucchini noodles, and spread them with all of the nut ricotta. Top that layer with the remaining eggplant noodles, and cover them with more tomato sauce. Sprinkle grated zucchini "cheese" and olives over the entire lasagna surface.

Cover the lasagna and refrigerate for at least a few hours to set. Cut into squares and serve.

THE "EATING IN THE RAW" CAESAR SALAD

1 garlic clove, chopped

2 heads organic romaine lettuce, chopped into bite-size pieces

DRESSING

½ cup grated raw-milk Pecorino Romano or Parmesan cheese

½ cup cold-pressed, extra-virgin olive oil

½ cup raw apple cider vinegar

1 fertile, organic egg

2 tablespoons Bragg Liquid Aminos

Juice of ½ lemon

SERVES 4

When I put this recipe in Eating in the Raw, *people loved it so much I knew I had to share it again. It's not vegan, but it is 100 percent raw, irresistibly tasty, and very nutritious. In fact, it could be a dinner all by itself.*

The ingredients are basically the same as a conventional Caesar salad but this raw version is, in my humble opinion, much better for you.

Crush the garlic clove and rub all over the inside of a large wooden salad bowl. Place the lettuce in the bowl.

In a medium mixing bowl, combine all the dressing ingredients. Add the dressing to the romaine lettuce in the salad bowl, and toss to combine.

HEATHY'S BANANA BERRY TART

CRUST

¼ cup dried apricots, soaked for 4 to 8 hours

½ cup Medjool dates, soaked for 4 to 8 hours

2 cups raw almonds, plus extra if needed

2 tablespoons ground flax seeds, plus extra if needed

1 to 2 tablespoons raw agave nectar, plus extra if needed

FILLING

4 fresh strawberries, sliced

6 to 8 ripe bananas, frozen

Fresh raspberries and fresh mint for garnish

TIP

Banana's high potassium, low salt combination makes it a tonic for controlling blood pressure. Increased potassium helps with concentration and enhances the ability to learn. The fiber in bananas (if they're ripe) helps normal, healthy bowel action.

SERVES 12; MAKES TWO 9-INCH TARTS

Be careful when choosing apricots to cook or eat. Most dried fruit is preserved with sulfuric acid, and they have coloring added to them. You want to find the best, cleanest, least-tampered-with apricots there are, and this goes for your other dried fruits as well. God didn't make apricots with artificial coloring, so why should you eat them with food dye?

For the crust, drain the apricots and dates and combine in a food processor with the almonds, flax seeds, and agave nectar. Pulse until the mixture comes together as a dough. If it is too sticky, add more almonds and flax; if it is too crumbly, add more agave nectar or some of the soaking liquid from the fruit. Press this dough into two 9-inch tart pans. Dehydrate at 105 degrees F until the entire surface of each tart crust is dry, 4 to 6 hours at least. Then lift the crust out of the pan, turn it over, and continue dehydrating until the entire crust is dry.

For the filling, arrange the sliced strawberries in the bottoms of the tart shells. Run the frozen bananas through a juicer and spoon the banana cream over the strawberries.

Serve immediately, garnished with fresh raspberries and mint leaves, or freeze the tarts until ready to serve. Let frozen tarts soften at room temperature for 10 minutes before garnishing and serving.

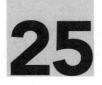

25 TERRA BELLA CAFE'S RAW "BARBECUE"

2 bell peppers, seeded and sliced

12 button mushrooms

12 grape tomatoes

1 onion, cut into 1-inch pieces

1 eggplant, cut into 1-inch cubes

MARINADE

1 cup cold-pressed, extra-virgin olive oil

2 tablespoons coconut oil

1 cup chopped red bell pepper

Juice of 2 limes

2 tablespoons grated ginger

2 teaspoons minced garlic

Himalayan salt to taste

1 cup packed fresh cilantro

BARBECUE SAUCE

2 cups diced fresh tomatoes

½ cup raisins, soaked until soft

1 cup sun-dried tomatoes, soaked until soft

1 cup chopped red onion

1 teaspoon ground cumin

Pinch of cayenne pepper

¼ cup chopped yellow onion

VEGGIE KEBABS WITH BARBECUE SAUCE

MAKES 4 KEBABS

Melissa Davison is an award-winner once again! Her kebabs and barbecue sauce won the Most Creative Yummy Dish over meat and cooked entries in the GrillMasters competition in Boise 2004! Congrats, Melissa! Your Terra Bella Cafe must be sprawling with people trying to get a taste of this award-winner!

Melissa has graciously shared this and the next three recipes.

Soak 4 wooden skewers in water for 30 minutes. Thread the vegetables on the skewers and arrange on a platter.

Mix the marinade ingredients, except the cilantro, in a blender until well combined. Add the cilantro and pulse once or twice to incorporate, but do not chop too fine. Pour over the kebabs and turn them to coat. Place kebabs in the dehydrator at 95 degrees F to warm and marinate for at least 2 hours.

For the sauce, if making, combine all the ingredients except the yellow onion in the blender and whir until well combined. Fold in the chopped onion. Brush liberally on the kebabs before placing in the dehydrator, saving some sauce for dipping or brushing on before serving.

JICA-RICE FRESH

1 large jicama, peeled

¼ cup finely chopped red onion

½ cup finely diced red bell pepper

½ cup finely diced yellow bell pepper

1 cup cherry tomatoes, halved

1 teaspoon minced garlic

⅛ teaspoon black pepper

1 tablespoon cold-pressed, extra-virgin olive oil

½ teaspoon ground cumin

¼ teaspoon Himalayan salt

2 tablespoons fresh lime juice, plus lime wedges for garnish

SERVES 4

Jicama is very versatile. Here it is in another signature Melissa Davison recipe served at Terra Bella Cafe. Many times my friends eat jicama and ask, "I thought you said this was raw food. Isn't this rice cooked?" Although some raw restaurants do serve rice, I love being able to tell my friends that they are not eating rice but a healthy, delicious vegetable!

Use a mandoline to cut the jicama into thin slices. Stack the sheets and cut into fine strips, then cut the strips crosswise to make ricelike pieces. Put the jicama "rice" in a mixing bowl. Add the remaining ingredients, except the lime wedges, and toss well to combine. Marinate at room temperature for 4 hours. Serve with lime wedges.

AVO-CORN STUFFED TOMATO

Ingredients

¼ cup sun-dried tomatoes, soaked until soft

3 cups chopped fresh tomatoes, plus 8 whole ripe tomatoes

1 tablespoon chili powder

1 tablespoon cold-pressed, extra-virgin olive oil

½ teaspoon Himalayan salt

3 cups sweet corn kernels

1 large firm avocado, pitted, peeled, and diced

½ cup fresh cilantro, chopped

1 tablespoon fresh lime juice

TIP

You could also stuff the mixture into seeded Anaheim peppers.

SERVES 8

This dish is just the perfect thing at a barbecue—a salad that doesn't look like one. It has enough vegetable ingredients to pass for a salad, but is stuffed in a tomato, not dumped on a plate; its presentation is actually something quite different and refreshing. While you're admiring this dish, notice how many servings of your five raw veggies or fruit you are getting!

Drain the sun-dried tomatoes and combine in the food processor with the fresh tomatoes, chili powder, olive oil, and salt. Pulse until combined.

In a bowl, mix together the corn, avocado, cilantro, and lime juice. Pour the tomato mixture over all, mix again, and set aside to marinate at room temperature for 10 to 20 minutes.

Core the whole tomatoes and use a melon scoop or a spoon to scoop out the seeds and soft flesh, leaving a hollowed-out shell. Fill with the corn-avocado-tomato mixture and serve.

MANGO DE FLAN

1 cup fresh mango, peeled, flesh removed from pit, and cubed

1 cup fresh coconut meat, preferably from a young Thai coconut

¼ cup almond milk

4 teaspoons raw agave syrup or honey

1 tablespoon coconut oil

Pinch of Himalayan salt

Soaked and drained Goji berries, and fresh mint sprigs for garnish

It's easy to tell if a mango is ripe: Roll the fruit between your fingers. If the skin gives just a little bit, then it's ripe. If it's mushy, it's overripe. Being overripe is not so bad, because the riper a fruit, the more enzymes and the sweeter it is. So it's up to you to decide whether you like tart fruit or sweet—it's all in the enzymes.

Coat three 6-inch Pyrex bowls with dark agave syrup. Set aside a few mango cubes for garnish. Combine the remaining ingredients in a blender or food processor, except the garnishes, and blend thoroughly until smooth.

Gently pour the mango mixture into three bowls. Set aside until the agave coating rises to the top of the mixture.

Smooth the surface gently without stirring in the agave coating. Place the bowls in the freezer for 30 minutes to set, but don't freeze completely. Invert the bowls onto dessert plates; the mango mixture should slide out. Garnish with fresh mango cubes, Goji berries, and mint.

26 DINER DINNER

MEATLESS MEAT LOAF

3 cups raw pecans, germinated (see pages 41–43)

3 cups raw walnuts, germinated

2 red bell peppers, seeded and chopped

1 cup chopped carrots

2 tablespoons paprika

1 tablespoon garlic powder

1 tablespoon poultry seasoning

Bragg Liquid Aminos or Nama Shoyu to taste

1 cup finely diced onion

1 cup finely diced celery

¼ cup chopped fresh parsley

Red Pepper Catsup (recipe follows) or Barbecue Sauce (page 126)

MAKES 1 LOAF

I saw a recipe like this in Juliano Brotman's book, Raw, and it was inspiring. When Kelly Serbonich told me she had a fabulous nut meat loaf recipe, I was dying to taste it. I loved meat loaf as a kid, and when I went raw, I didn't want to give it up. Kelly's is great-tasting and easy to make.

The most time-consuming part of the recipe is germinating the nuts properly, since not every nut germinates at the same speed. (See the germination chart on page 43.)

In a mixing bowl, combine the pecans, walnuts, bell pepper, carrot, paprika, garlic powder, poultry seasoning, and Bragg Liquid Aminos and mix well. Process this mixture through the Jack LaLanne juicer using the homogenizing attachment, or process in your food processor. Season with Bragg Liquid Aminos or Nama Shoyu and transfer to a large bowl. Add the onion, celery, and parsley and use your hands to mix thoroughly.

Form the mixture into a loaf shape and place on a Teflex-lined dehydrator tray. Dehydrate 8 to 12 hours, using the dehydrator as you might a Crock-Pot. Top with Red Pepper Catsup several hours before serving and return to the dehydrator for 2 to 3 more hours. Slice and serve with catsup or barbecue sauce.

red pepper catsup   MAKES 2 CUPS

"Mayo! Catsup! What's next?" you might be thinking. "I thought this book was about raw food, and I was going to be starving and sucking on carrots." Well, not unless you want to suck on carrots, which is your perfect right. It is still somewhat of a free country.

I saw a History Channel documentary on catsup, which described how the catsup industry originally used all the rotten pieces of the tomato and added toxic substances to kill the tart, rotten taste, prompting the newly formed FDA to pass a law requiring companies to list every ingredient in their products. In the nineteenth century, catsup had so many toxins, people were falling ill, all this from what was basically a pureed tomato. Thank goodness for the FDA; thank goodness for Kelly Serbonich's recipe!

2 cups chopped red bell pepper

¼ cup chopped red onion

⅛ cup chopped red beet

2 tablespoons paprika

2 tablespoons ground flax seeds

1 tablespoon celery powder (optional, see Tip)

2 teaspoons garlic powder

Pinch of ground cloves

⅔ cup cold-pressed, extra-virgin olive oil

1½ tablespoons fresh lemon juice

¼ teaspoon raw agave nectar

Bragg Liquid Aminos or Nama Shoyu to taste

Combine all the catsup ingredients in the blender, except the Bragg Liquid Aminos or Nama Shoyu. Blend well and season with Bragg Liquid Aminos or Nama Shoyu.

TIP
You can make your own celery powder by dehydrating celery, then grinding it to a powder with a spice or coffee grinder.

CABBAGE AND PEAS WITH TARRAGON

2 cups fresh shelled peas

2 cups diced green and/or red cabbage

½ cup chopped fresh parsley

⅓ cup diced red onion

1 tablespoon dried tarragon

DRESSING

1 cup cold-pressed, extra-virgin olive oil

1 tablespoon dried tarragon

2¼ teaspoons fresh lemon juice

1 teaspoon dry mustard

Pinch of cayenne pepper

1 garlic clove

2 teaspoons Bragg Liquid Aminos or Nama Shoyu

¼ cup purified water

SERVES 8

A great thing about raw recipes is that they are so flexible. If you decide to leave out an ingredient that you don't like, the soufflé won't collapse, figuratively speaking. So if you want to leave one or two ingredients out of this recipe from Kelly Serbonich, you won't kill it. Play around with it, experiment, and enjoy eating your mistakes.

Combine the peas, cabbage, parsley, onion, and tarragon in a mixing bowl.

Combine the dressing ingredients in a blender and whir until well combined. Taste for seasoning and add more Bragg Liquid Aminos if necessary.

Pour the dressing over the salad mixture, mix gently, and marinate at room temperature for at least 30 minutes before serving.

CHRISSY'S APPLE PIE WITH WHIPPED CREAM

Raw carob powder for sprinkling pie plate

2 cups raw almonds

40 pitted dates, soaked for 1 hour and drained

2 apples, 1 cored and chopped and the other thinly sliced and dehydrated at 115 degrees F for 2 to 4 hours

1 teaspoon ground cinnamon

½ teaspoon nutmeg

¼ teaspoon Himalayan salt

Kelly's Macadamia Whipped Cream (recipe follows, optional)

SERVES 8

When my sister Christine and I are sitting around, guiltlessly eating apple pie with whipped cream, it's as though we're kids again. This is her raw version of a beloved American classic.

Grease the bottom of a 9-inch pie plate with a little cold-pressed olive oil and dust with raw carob powder; this will keep the piecrust from sticking to the pie plate. To make the piecrust, combine the almonds and 10 of the dates in the food processor and chop until coarsely ground and starting to form a ball. Press the dough evenly into the bottom of the pie plate and up the sides.

Combine the remaining 30 dates, chopped apple, cinnamon, nutmeg, and salt in the food processor. Process until the mixture is smooth and caramel-like. Pour the filling into the prepared piecrust. Arrange the dehydrated apple slices on top.

Serve with Kelly's Macadamia Whipped Cream on the side, if desired.

kelly's macadamia whipped cream

I said you can make whipped cream without using raw dairy cream, and here's how. I included this recipe from Kelly Serbonich in Eating in the Raw, *but it goes so well with apple pie, I didn't want you to miss out. We have a recipe for "real" dairy whipped cream on page 75—make them both and decide which you prefer. You may like 'em both, you never know.*

The first time I saw a raw, vegan whipped cream recipe in Juliano Brotman's book, Raw, *I said out loud, "I am a real whipped cream lover. You're telling me you can make cream with orange juice that tastes like whipped cream? You have got to be kidding me." Well, I ate my words. I eat them nearly every day.*

1 cup macadamia nuts, soaked for 8 to 10 hours and dehydrated at 115 degrees F for 12 hours

½ cup fresh, young coconut water (see Tip, page 97)

5 pitted dates, soaked for 2 hours and drained

1 tablespoon organic, cold-pressed coconut butter

Combine all the ingredients in a blender and whir until smooth and creamy. Chill for at least 1 hour before serving.

TIP

My sister and I noticed that this cream whips best in the Vita-Mix blender. I think the blades move faster and aerate the nut cream more than most other blenders, making the cream lighter.

27 SPRING FLING MENU

THREE-NUT PESTO PASTA

4 medium zucchini

2 cherry tomatoes, quartered

6 asparagus stalks, thinly sliced on an angle

½ cup chopped fresh cilantro

PESTO

2 cups raw pine nuts

½ cup raw cashews

½ cup raw macadamia nuts

4 garlic cloves, minced

6 tablespoons fresh lemon juice

4 teaspoons Himalayan salt

TIP

The sauce alone makes a fabulous dip, and you can add whatever vegetables you want to the zucchini.

SERVES 6

Once a month, Lisa Montgomery sponsors a raw food potluck dinner in the Philadelphia area that draws people from several hours away. She acts as hostess and publishes the participants' recipes in a monthly newsletter. As if that's not enough, Lisa's talented in the kitchen as well.

I cannot count how many times people have told me that the one thing they could not give up if they went raw is pasta. They obviously haven't tried Lisa's pesto pasta! It's simple, easy, healthy, and reminds me of regular pasta, but, honestly, it tastes even better!

Many of the recipes in this book come from people who participate in Lisa's monthly get-together. Thank you, Lisa, for introducing me to them.

Use a spiral slicer to cut the zucchini into long strips and put in a serving bowl. Add the tomatoes, asparagus, and cilantro.

Combine the pine nuts, cashews, macadamia nuts, garlic, lemon juice, and salt in a food processor and process until smooth and saucelike. Pour the sauce over the vegetables and toss well.

BABY SPINACH SALAD WITH CARROT HORSERADISH DRESSING

DRESSING

2 large carrots, coarsely chopped

1 or 2 celery stalks, coarsely chopped

2 tablespoons raw apple cider vinegar

1 tablespoon minced fresh gingerroot, or more to taste

2 teaspoons freshly grated horseradish, or more to taste

1 to 2 apples, sliced

3 cups baby spinach leaves

If you love the burn you feel in your mouth and nose when you eat something spicy, then you'll love this dressing. Fresh horseradish root is pungent and can be grown in your garden. My brother-in-law Bill grows his own, and he makes the best horseradish—and KellyAnn Palazzolo makes the best horseradish dressing.

Combine the dressing ingredients in a blender and blend till smooth. If the dressing seems too thick, add some purified water. Adjust the ginger or horseradish as desired.

Put the spinach and apples in a bowl and pour the dressing over them. Toss and serve.

BANANA TRIFLE

BANANA LAYER

8 ripe bananas

¼ cup raw agave nectar

2 tablespoons coconut oil

CASHEW LAYER

2½ cups raw cashews

½ cup date sugar

CINNAMON LAYER

6 tablespoons raw carob powder, sifted

3 tablespoons date sugar

1½ tablespoons cinnamon

Banana slices for garnish (optional)

TIP

If you find it difficult to spread the banana layer on top of the cashew layer, place the trifle bowl in the freezer for a short time after adding each cashew layer.

This is another Christine Alt concoction, and it is great. The only drawback is that you have to eat it within a few hours of making it. Left overnight, even in a refrigerator, the trifle becomes mushy and unappetizing. But hey, eating it all in one shot shouldn't be too much of a hardship, should it?

For the banana layer, in a mixing bowl, mash the bananas with a fork or potato masher. Stir in the agave nectar and coconut oil. (If you prefer a smoother texture, blend the ingredients in a blender.) Set aside.

For the cashew layer, grind the cashews and date sugar in a food processor, blender, or coffee grinder until well ground. The mixture should be coarse. Set aside.

Mix all the ingredients for the cinnamon layer in a small bowl.

In a trifle bowl (or individual parfait glasses), spread one-third of the cashew layer evenly over the bottom. Carefully pour or spoon one-third of the banana cream over the cashew layer. Sprinkle with one-third of the cinnamon layer. Repeat the layers 2 more times. Top with banana slices if you like. Refrigerate about 2 hours or until firm.

28 COMFORT FOOD DINNER

BROCCOLI CHEDDAR CANNELLONI

TOMATO SAUCE TOPPING

½ cup sun-dried tomatoes, soaked for 2 hours

¼ cup purified water

½ teaspoon fresh lemon juice

1 tablespoon cold-pressed, extra-virgin olive oil

1 garlic clove

1 tablespoon fresh thyme or oregano

2 medium tomatoes, chopped

½ cup chopped fresh basil

¼ cup fresh oregano leaves

½ teaspoon Himalayan salt

SERVES 4

Dan Hoyt—Raw Chef Dan—is a master at creating unbelievable raw foods. And this one you have to taste to believe.

Again, in place of pasta we use a veggie. And again, I say that pasta has no flavor—it's basically wallpaper paste. Veggies have mild flavors that distinguish one from another. They also take on the flavor of heavier spices, and in this case, a tomato sauce. This is an easy sauce to make. It doesn't burn your stomach, and you may wonder why nobody told you about it before you got hooked on your acid indigestion meds. At least try it; I think you'll like it.

For the sauce, blend the sun-dried tomatoes, water, lemon juice, olive oil, and thyme in a blender until smooth. Transfer to the bowl of a food processor and add the fresh tomatoes, basil, fresh oregano, and salt. Pulse until the ingredients are well combined into a thick, coarse sauce (do not puree). Set aside.

FILLING

2 broccoli stalks (with the crowns), cut into chunks

1 teaspoon grated nutmeg

1 tablespoon chopped fresh rosemary

1 tablespoon chopped fresh sage

½ cup raw cashews, soaked for 2 hours

½ cup sunflower seeds, sprouted (see pages 41–43)

¼ cup fresh lemon juice

½ tablespoon salt

CANNELLONI "SHELLS"

1 large zucchini

¼ cup raw pine nuts for garnish

To make the filling, finely chop the broccoli in the food processor. Add the nutmeg and rosemary and process until incorporated. Transfer the broccoli to a mixing bowl and, without washing out the work bowl, combine the sage, cashews, sunflower sprouts, lemon juice, and salt in the food processor; process until smooth. Stir the cashew mixture into the broccoli until well blended and set aside.

Use a mandoline or vegetable peeler to shave long wide strips from the zucchini; these will be your cannelloni "shells." Place 4 of the strips side by side, overlapping a bit, to make a square mat of sliced zucchini. Place a few tablespoons of the broccoli mixture along one long edge and roll the mixture in the zucchini slices to create a long filled tube. Repeat with the remaining zucchini strips and filling. Serve in a pool of tomato sauce. Top with a little more tomato sauce and pine nuts.

SPICED SQUASH

½ cup chopped sun-dried tomato, soaked for 2 hours and drained

2 tablespoons cold-pressed, extra-virgin olive oil

1 tablespoon minced white onion

1 tablespoon minced fresh oregano

1 tablespoon minced fresh basil

1 tablespoon minced fresh dill

1 tablespoon minced fresh sage

1 teaspoon Himalayan salt

2 zucchini, sliced

2 yellow summer squash, sliced

SERVES 4

Marinating makes all the difference in the world for some dishes, and this recipe is no exception. According to Raw Chef Dan Hoyt, in this spiced squash he created, the more you marinate, the better those veggies can absorb the spices and the tastier they will be. If you want a milder flavor, marinate them for less time.

In a mixing bowl, combine the sun-dried tomatoes, oil, onion, chopped fresh herbs, and salt. Add the sliced squash and toss to coat. Marinate for 2 hours before serving.

QUINTESSENCE VANILLA PUDDING WITH FRESH BERRIES

1 large ripe smooth-skinned (not Hass) avocado, chilled

1 tablespoon high-quality vanilla extract

2 tablespoons raw agave nectar or raw honey

½ teaspoon Himalayan salt

⅔ cup chilled purified water

4 large fresh strawberries, hulled and sliced, or 1 mango, chopped

SERVES 4

Here we go with the avocados again. When I take people to Quintessence restaurant, I don't tell them that the pudding or mousse is made with avocados until after they have tasted it. If I told them before, chances are they wouldn't try it. Once I've told them, well, most people are pleasantly surprised. At least this is what they tell me as they're finishing off their pudding. Come on, what are you waiting for, an invitation?

Pit and peel the avocado and put in a blender. Add the vanilla, agave or honey, salt, and water and whir until smooth.

Serve in a wide bowl, topped with fresh strawberries and/or chopped mango.

29

PEPPER AND SALAD DINNER

½ cup dried pineapple

½ dried mango

4 cups raw cashews, soaked for 2 hours and drained

2 cups raw macadamia nuts, soaked for 2 hours and drained

1 cup whole cherry tomatoes

2 cups chopped red or yellow bell peppers, plus 6 whole peppers

½ cup diced avocado

1¾ cups chopped fresh mango

2¼ cups chopped fresh cilantro

¼ cup snipped fresh chives

2½ teaspoons raw agave nectar

1 teaspoon ground cumin

1 teaspoon dried and ground pomegranate seeds

¾ cup diced plum tomatoes

1 teaspoon habanero pepper (optional)

½ cup chopped red onions

2 teaspoons Himalayan salt

BELIVE MOM'S STUFFED BELL PEPPERS

SERVES 6

Brian Lucas goes by the name Chef BeLive Light, and he is very talented. You may find this recipe a little more challenging than many of the others in this book. But give it a try. It just may be easier than you think, and it's definitely worth it! Think of it as a tribute. You're making Mom's stuffed peppers—only raw—and the effort is worth it.

When blending these ingredients, use a high-powered blender such as a Vita-Mix. Seems that every chef I asked uses it!

In separate bowls, soak ¼ cup of the dried pineapple and ¼ cup of the dried mango in purified water to cover for 60 minutes. Drain and set aside the soaking water. Chop the remaining dried pineapple and dried mango.

In a blender or food processor, combine the cashews, macadamia nuts, whole cherry tomatoes, 1 cup of the chopped bell pepper, the avocado, the soaked dried pineapple and mango, ¼ cup of the chopped fresh mango 1¼ cups of the cilantro, the chives, agave, cumin, pomegranate seeds, and optional habanero pepper. Pulse the mixture to chop and combine it. Then add ½ cup each of the reserved pineapple and mango soaking water (discard the rest). Process until smooth and liquid.

In a separate large mixing bowl, combine the remaining 1½ cups of chopped fresh mango, the remaining 1 cup of chopped bell pepper, the diced tomatoes, and red onions. Toss to mix, then pour the blended mixture over all and toss again to coat thoroughly.

Cut the whole peppers in half, remove the seeds, then stuff them with the filling. Sprinkle with the remaining chopped cilantro, the diced dried mango, diced dried pineapple, and Himalayan salt and serve.

CHOPPED SPINACH SALAD WITH ESSENTIAL DRESSING

ESSENTIAL DRESSING

¼ cup flax seed oil or hemp oil

¼ cup Bragg Liquid Aminos (or purified water)

Dash of organic dried parsley flakes and/or other seasoning, such as kelp flakes, to taste

SALAD

10 to 12 ounces spinach leaves, torn into bite-size pieces

½ cup small cauliflower florets, coarsely chopped

2 celery stalks, chopped

2 shallots or 1 small red onion, chopped

½ cup chopped fresh basil

2 red bell peppers, seeded and chopped

¼ cup raw pine nuts

SERVES 6

I know this recipe involves a lot of chopping, but I find that the more you chop these ingredients, the tastier the salad. Just make sure you don't go overboard. You don't want mush. (See page 81 for information on spinach.)

Combine all the dressing ingredients in a bowl and whisk to blend.

For the salad, in a large bowl, combine all the ingredients but the pine nuts and mix well. Sprinkle the pine nuts on top. Drizzle with the dressing, toss again, and serve.

VITO NATALE'S FRUIT AND CHOCOLATE DECADENCE

1 cup chocolate

1 cup raw agave nectar

1 cup raw carob powder

¾ cup coconut oil

1 tablespoon raw sesame seeds

½ cup raw almonds, germinated (see pages 41–43)

1 cup raw cashews, germinated (see pages 41–43)

1 cup purified water

Seasonal fresh berries of your choice (if using strawberries, hull and slice)

Fresh mint leaves for garnish

Kelly's Macadamia Whipped Cream (optional, page 134)

TIP

Raw chocolate? Sure! Raw organic cacao nibs are bits of dried cacao beans. They are not processed in any way. Hard pieces can be powdered in a coffee grinder.

SERVES 12

What can I say about chocolate that you don't already know? How about that Vito Natale's dessert is just about the chocolatiest, most amazing dessert ever? Don't take my word for it. Make it. It's not called "decadence" for nothing!

Combine the chocolate, agave, carob, coconut oil, sesame seeds, and germinated almonds in a blender and whir until very smooth; transfer to a mixing bowl and set aside.

Clean out the blender, then add the cashews and water and blend until the mixture is smooth and creamy. Fold into the chocolate mixture, until it is very smooth.

Spoon the mixture into a square baking dish, preferably glass, and smooth the top. Refrigerate for 1 hour or more. Cut into squares, remove from the dish, and serve topped with sliced or whole berries and mint leaves. Add a dollop of whipped cream if desired.

30

SUSHI SAMBA
SUMMER

1 small watermelon

½ pound daikon radish, chopped

10 cucumbers, 5 peeled and chopped, 5 unpeeled and finely diced

4 coarsely chopped shallots

1 fresh gingerroot knob, peeled and chopped

¼ cup Namu Shoyu

¼ cup cold-pressed, extra virgin olive oil

1 bunch fresh mint, stems removed and leaves chopped

1 red onion, finely diced

Himalayan salt to taste

Freshly ground white pepper to taste

2 fresh limes

CHILLED
WATERMELON SOUP

SERVES 8

I never thought I would say "watermelon" and "daikon radish" in the same sentence. But, hey, you're in the raw-food world now and the rules were made to be broken. Take the adage that fats are fattening. Maybe in the cooked world they are, but in the raw world, I eat fats to boost my immune system and keep my skin looking as young as possible for as long as possible.

Scoop out the sweet flesh from the watermelon rind, removing as many seeds as possible. In a blender, combine the watermelon, daikon radish, chopped peeled cucumbers, shallots, ginger, Namu Shoyu, and olive oil and puree on high speed for at least 3 minutes, or until all the ingredients liquefy. (You may have to do this in two or more batches.) Chill for at least 8 hours, then pass it through a fine-mesh sieve. Discard all solids.

In a small bowl mix the mint, red onion, and diced cucumber. Season this mixture with salt and pepper.

To serve, spoon the watermelon broth into large chilled bowls, spoon a dollop of the cucumber, mint, and onion mixture in the center, and finish with a squeeze of lime.

SASHIMI CEVICHE

SERVES 1

1 tablespoon fresh
orange juice

1 teaspoon fresh lemon juice

1 teaspoon fresh lime juice

1 teaspoon Namu Shoyu

⅛ teaspoon aji amarillo
paste (see Note)

¼ teaspoon grated fresh
gingerroot

Pinch of Himalayan salt

2 tablespoons cold-pressed,
extra-virgin olive oil, plus
extra for drizzling on a dish

¼ pound sashimi-grade tuna

1 tablespoon julienned
red onion

1 tablespoon julienned
yellow bell pepper

1 tablespoon julienned
celery

4 thin slices of jalapeño

1 cherry tomato, quartered

⅛ teaspoon minced chives

Sushi Samba is not a raw restaurant, but maybe that's part of the reason why I like eating there. I can choose things from the same menu everyone else uses and always find something that satisfies my mood. Not only that, with the exception of an occasional condiment or minor ingredient, I can eat entirely raw.

One summer I lived on Michael Cressotti's delicious ceviche. You don't feel too full when you stand up from the table, yet it stays with you and you're not hungry an hour later. It makes you feel satisfied but light—perfect for the summer.

I love it in the winter, too. It's full of essential oils that burn off cleanly and keep you warm. Clearly, it's wonderful anytime!

In a glass mixing bowl, combine the citrus juices, Namu Shoyu, aji amarillo paste, ginger, and salt. Slowly drizzle in the oil while whisking briskly. Set aside.

Slice the fish thinly across the grain into 4 slices.

In a separate glass bowl, combine the fish, onion, bell pepper, celery, jalapeño, and tomatoes.

Add the citrus and oil to the fish and vegetables and toss. Place the ceviche on a serving plate, drizzle with oil, and sprinkle chives over the presentation for garnish.

NOTE: Aji amarillo paste is a spicy pepper sauce that is commonly used in Latin American dishes. You won't find it in health-food stores, but it is available online. Like a few other ingredients in The Raw 50, it is not raw. It's included here because there is only a tiny quantity in the recipe, and its unique, zesty taste is delicious. But you can make this recipe—not the Sushi Samba way—with raw spices to add a different sort of zest. It's your choice.

TIP

You can use other sashimi-grade fish, like salmon. Tell your fish supplier that you are not cooking it, so you get the freshest fish he has.

SHAVED ASPARAGUS SALAD

SERVES 2

10 asparagus spears

1 small carrot

1 small daikon radish

2 red radishes

3 plum tomatoes

¼ cup raw apple cider vinegar

¼ cup Udo's Choice oil blend

Salt and pepper to taste

2 shiso leaves

Trim off the ends of the asparagus, about 1 inch from the bottom and discard. With a vegetable peeler in hand, hold each asparagus and shave downward along the stem to make long strips, avoiding the top. Toss the strips into a salad bowl. Dice the tops and toss them in the bowl.

Peel the carrot and daikon radish, then make strips with the vegetable peeler just as you did with the asparagus, and toss them in the bowl.

Using a mandoline, slice the common radishes paper-thin and add to the bowl.

In a blender, pulse together the tomatoes, vinegar, oil, salt, and pepper. Pass this mixture through a fine-mesh sieve and chill.

Combine the blended salad dressing with the vegetables in the salad bowl and toss lightly. Serve in separate bowls atop a shiso leaf.

VITO'S FROZEN WATERMELON CHEESECAKE

1 young Thai coconut

2 cups raw cashews

2 tablespoons raw agave nectar

2 tablespoons raw honey

Pinch of Himalayan salt

1 teaspoon raw sesame seeds

¼ cup purified water

1 cup cubed and seeded watermelon

½ cup raw chopped almonds for garnish (optional)

Kiwi slices for garnish (optional)

SERVES 8

Usually, I like a watermelon sorbet; it is light and easy (in the sorbet recipe on page 102 you can substitute watermelon for the raspberry). But if you are having company, you may want to surprise and please them with a cake they can eat guilt free.

Open the coconut (see Tip, page 97) and pour out ½ cup of coconut water; save or discard the rest. Pry out the coconut meat and measure ¼ cup, reserving the rest for another use.

Place the coconut water and meat in a blender or food processor. Add the agave nectar, honey, salt, sesame seeds, water, and watermelon, and process until thoroughly combined. Scrape the mixture into a glass pie dish and place in the freezer for at least 1 hour until firm.

Cut into wedges and serve garnished with a sprinkle of chopped almonds and a few kiwi slices if desired.

TIP

Watermelon is an excellent source of vitamins A and C as well as B_6 and B_1, carotenoid lycopene, magnesium, and potassium. Its seeds, being of fat and protein, are edible—and so is the rind!

GINGER TANSEN

CERVICAL CANCER AND SINUS PROBLEM

Modesto, California

No one wants to hear the word cancer—especially not someone in her twenties.

Ginger's stepfather died of colon cancer in 2001 at the age of forty-three. In 2002, her grandfather lost his battle with lung cancer. Then, just a year later, her grandmother succumbed to the same disease.

"I never imagined so many people in my life, so many people I was close to and loved, would die in such a short period of time," she recalls sadly.

Shortly after her grandmother's death, Ginger went for her annual gynecological exam. The doctor did a Pap smear, Ginger went home, and she didn't think twice about it. When no one called her with the results, she assumed everything was normal. But a few months later, when she called her gynecologist's office, the receptionist put her on hold. Then the doctor got on the line.

"We need to see you right away," the doctor said. Somehow they had failed to inform her that her test results were anything but normal. Ginger had stage III cervical cancer, which has about a 50 percent five-year survival rate. She needed surgery, the doctor said, and soon.

"When I heard the word 'cancer' I freaked out and everything in my life changed," Ginger says. She resolved she was not going to be the fourth member of her family to die of the disease. Her doctor performed a loop electrosurgical excision procedure, known as a LEEP, to surgically remove the cancerous cells. But it was only partially successful, and following the procedure, Ginger had a series of infections. "I had nothing but problems after that small surgery," she says, "and there were still cancerous cells.

"I decided that even though the cancer wasn't all gone, I wanted to have them watch it for a while before they went back in to do more cutting. In the meantime whatever it took to get well, I was going to do it," Ginger says.

Ginger set out to learn all she could about what she could do to improve her health. She read and read. "I started doing my own research into the effect of diet on health. I knew that what I ate could make a real difference, so first I became a vegetarian, then a vegan. Then one day I spotted an article about Carol Alt and raw food. It mentioned a book she had written that explained how eating raw food helped restore good health. I knew who Carol was, so I ordered it. I got *Eating in the Raw,* read it, and then I read it again and again. When Carol wrote about her sinus problems and how eating raw cured her sinus infections, she could have been talking to me; I had sinus problems at least seven times a year," Ginger says.

Ginger bought more books about raw food. "The more I read, the more I knew that eating raw food could be answer to my health problems."

So Ginger bought a juicer and "juiced like crazy," she says. She made recipes out of *Eating in the Raw* and before long, saw real changes in her health.

"My sinus problems simply stopped. Finally, I could breathe!" she says.

But that was just the beginning.

After her surgery, Ginger's doctor had set her up on a schedule of testing every three months to keep an eye on the cancerous cells. In June 2005, less than a year and half after her surgery and barely half a year since going raw, she returned to the gynecologist for a biopsy to check on the cells' progress. The doctor was intending to take another biopsy, but what he saw didn't make sense. The cancerous cells seemed to have disappeared—and his test showed that the cancer was simply gone.

"I changed what I was eating. That is what was different. That's it. I was eating raw," Ginger recalls.

Since that first clean bill of health, Ginger has returned to the doctor regularly and remains cancer free. She has noticed other, subtler changes as well.

"Eating raw just makes me feel better. My inner self is somehow different. I'm more compassionate toward others, to children, to animals. I find I want to help others, and not just keep up with the Joneses. I'm more spiritual, more connected to my church. My outlook on life has changed. I cherish life," Ginger says.

And cherish it she should. Not yet thirty, it seems Ginger has a long, healthy life ahead to make the most of.

10 RAW
DRINKS

One of the most positive developments I have seen in the food world in the past five years is the proliferation of juice bars. Not that Dunkin' Donuts is likely to be displaced by Jamba Juice any time soon, **but juices, smoothies, and other healthy drinks are certainly in fashion and much easier to come by than ever before.** However, not all smoothies and juice drinks are created equal. In fact, some are so packed with sugar and calories, you might as well be drinking a milk shake! Avoid those drinks containing pasteurized milk, yogurt, cream, or bottled juice. (Yes, most juices are pasteurized. If they don't squeeze it in front of you, I would be suspicious!)

Of course, the best way to know exactly what is in your raw drink is to make it yourself. Fortunately, it is easy and fun to make raw drinks, and once you've invested in a good-quality juicer (see page 24), you're pretty much set to make any kind of raw drink you can dream up.

This book could have been all about raw drinks. The possibilities are endless. A raw drink can be a treat or a meal in itself, and you can enjoy them sitting around with friends or on the go. They're refreshing and packed with nutrition, and are a great way to get your daily dose of fruit or veggies. Done right, how could you not enjoy a raw drink?

Jack LaLanne is the original American health and fitness guru. While most people know him as a fitness expert, he has also been trying to get people to eat more raw food for more than half a century. He insists that eating five servings of raw vegetables and five servings of raw fruit each day has been key to his own vitality and longevity.

Jack believes in juicing and so do I. You don't need to juice to benefit from eating raw. But the benefits of making fresh, raw juices are hard to overstate. Juices are refreshing. You get a lot of nutrients in quick-and-easy form. You can combine flavors that otherwise are impossible to blend together. And some foods actually need to be juiced to get their maximum benefit. Some people don't realize, for example, that just eating a raw carrot without juicing it barely gets any of its precious beta-carotene into your system because chewing simply doesn't break down the cellulose walls. But juicing does. And even if the thought of carrot juice doesn't appeal to your palate, combined with apple juice, for example, it's simply delicious.

In his nineties now, Jack LaLanne and his wife, Elaine, are still going strong and still helping people. The first recipe is one of Jack's own favorites. I limited the selection here to ten, but you certainly don't need to stop there. Use these suggestions to get you started; then whip up your own signature blends!

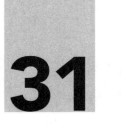

31 JACK LALANNE'S ENERGY BOOST

1 carrot, trimmed

1 celery stalk with leaves

1 beet with roots and leaves, scrubbed

Small handful of fresh parsley leaves

3 to 4 lettuce leaves

Small bunch of watercress

Small handful of spinach leaves

3 tomatoes, halved

Salt to taste

SERVES 1

I did an infomercial with Jack LaLanne, and he told me that he has an Energy Boost drink nearly every day. I thought, "Yeah, right, as if this guy needs any more energy!" Apparently it works!

One by one, feed the vegetables into the juicer, cutting the carrot, celery and beet into pieces if necessary to fit through the feed tube. Roll the greens like a cigar in a paper towel to remove any excess water from washing them, and then push them through the feed tube. Stir the juice and enjoy!

32 QUINTESSENCE VANILLA AVOCADO MILK

¼ ripe avocado

½ teaspoon high-quality vanilla extract

⅛ teaspoon Himalayan salt

1 tablespoon raw agave nectar or raw honey

1½ cups purified water, as needed (optional)

½ cup crushed ice (optional)

TIP

Remember to put your avocados into a brown paper bag and into a dark cupboard to ripen them. But don't forget they're there, which I've done more than once, and boy, what a mess. Now, I put a note on the cupboard door to remind myself to check on the avocados.

SERVES 1

The great thing about this drink is that it's not just sweet. Many people like to start their day with something sweet, such as a piece of fruit, a muffin, or a bagel. (Yes, that wheat flour in the bagel is a simple carbohydrate, otherwise known as a simple sugar.) But sweet things like fruit don't feed the body what it needs to function over a long period of time. Sugar in any form is used up quickly and has a glycemic effect—it makes your pancreas produce insulin. That wouldn't be bad if the insulin was kept at a constant level. But with a fruit or wheat sugar spike in the morning, and with no solid follow up, you're left tired or hungry about an hour later.

So, what should you do? With a drink like this, you not only have the sugar you need for instant energy, you also have the fats from the raw avocado that are clean burning and come with their own enzymes. The fats become an energy source later in the morning. That way, you're not left hungry after the sugar burns off; you are left with the energy from the fats, meaning you're well fed all morning long.

Combine the avocado, vanilla, salt, and agave nectar in a blender and puree. Add as much of the purified water as needed and continue to whir until smooth. Pour over ice, if you wish, and serve.

33 SWEET LEMON-LIME ORANGEADE

2 cups purified water

Juice of 1 lemon

Juice of 1 lime

Raw agave nectar to taste

2 orange slices

SERVES 2 TO 3

This drink is 100 percent fruit juice, so I always suggest mixing it with water. I feel you should never just drink straight fruit juice because it contains too much sugar.

Pour the water into a pitcher and stir in the lemon and lime juice. Add in agave nectar to achieve desired sweetness. Add the orange slices and ice, if desired, and stir and serve.

34 FOUNTAIN OF YOUTH SWEET CUCUMBER SUMMER JUICE

1 celery stalk

1 large cucumber, peeled

1 red or yellow bell pepper

½ sweet red apple or ripe pear

SERVES 1

You need five servings each of raw fruit and veggies every day, and you get four servings out of ten right here. My friend John Moretti at Fountain of Youth in Westport, Connecticut, makes this drink for me. It is quick, easy to make, and so healthy. (See my tip on cucumbers on page 92.)

Feed all the ingredients through the juicer. Stir well and serve.

35 ALMOND MILK, TWO WAYS

CHEATER'S ALMOND NUT MILK

SERVES 1

2 tablespoons smooth raw almond butter

1 cup purified water

Raw honey or agave nectar (optional)

I call this "cheater's" almond milk because you don't have to germinate your almonds, grind them in the blender, or filter out the almond bits; it is all done for you by Marantha, the company that makes raw almond butter.

Blend the almond butter and water in a blender or food processor, adding honey or a drop of agave if desired. Shake it again. Mmm!

For a delicious raisin flavor combine the almond milk with 7 raisins; whir in the blender to combine.

TIP

Nut milk lasts several days in the fridge, and longer if vacuum sealed. Gently shake it to remix before using.

LIVE LIVE'S ALMOND NUT MILK

SERVES 1

1 cup almonds or nut of your choice, germinated (see pages 41–43)

3 to 5 cups purified water

1 tablespoon raw agave nectar or raw honey

This is the way Christopher from "live live & organic" taught me to make it from scratch!

Combine the germinated nuts and water in the blender and whir until the nuts are practically pulverized. Strain through cheesecloth and discard the solids. Return the liquid to the blender, add the agave nectar or honey, and whir.

36 DAVID JUBB'S GINGER WARMER

2 inches fresh gingerroot, peeled

½ cinnamon stick

4 cups purified water

2 slices lemon

TIP

Cinnamon is very high in antioxidants, and the oil of cinnamon has antimicrobial properties. Over the years, it has been used to treat diarrhea and digestive problems, but newscientist.com reports that in studies just ½ teaspoon a day seemed to significantly reduce blood sugar levels and the levels of fats and "bad" cholesterol in the blood.

SERVES 2

Dr. David Jubb is known for his advice on health, but he also makes and sells great food. In fact, he is one of the original great raw chefs.

This is a great-tasting drink. But it is also somewhat medicinal: Got indigestion? Ate cooked food? Ginger really settles the stomach. Lemon is very alkalinizing, which settles the body and the mind alike. Put it all together, and maybe this is something you should take right before bed.

To learn more about David Jubb, go to jubbs-longevity.com.

Mince the gingerroot, grate it, or press through a garlic press. Combine the minced ginger, cinnamon stick, and water in a small pan and heat until warm, but well below the boiling point. Pour through a strainer into two cups. Serve with a slice of lemon.

37 PENNI'S PERFECT GREEN GODDESS

1 bunch kale or spinach

3 celery stalks

1 lemon, peeled

1 bunch parsley

1 fresh gingerroot knob, peeled

1 apple, any variety

TIP

You can play with the taste by changing the kind of apple you use. Granny Smith makes the drink tart, while Fuji or Braeburn apples make for a sweeter drink. It's all a matter of preference.

SERVES 1

It's my experience that many people shy away from vegetable juices because they think of them as medicine. They think "I have to take my veggie juice, I have to take my veggie juice . . ." Because these people are thinking medicinally, they try to cram as many veggies into one juice as they can. Even if they're getting maximum benefit, they are probably finding minimum taste. Some veggies just don't taste good together. Not so with Penni Shelton's Green Goddess. This really is the perfect mixture of greens. It will make you a goddess! Or at the very least, it will put a smile on your face while being very good for you—unlike any medicine you ever tasted before.

Feed all the ingredients through your juicer. Stir well and serve.

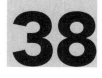

38 THE SHELTON (A NOT-SO-GREEN DRINK)

1 frozen banana

Handful of strawberries

½ cup fresh almond milk (page 158)

Juice of 1 orange

Splash of agave nectar

2 tablespoons Crystal Manna flakes

TIP

Bananas contain the protein tryptophan, a natural mood enhancer that can also help you to relax. When it converts to serotonin, tryptophan can not only help lift depression but also make you feel good all over.

SERVES 1

This is another of Tulsa-based Penni Shelton's creations. It's her favorite green drink, though it's not as green as others as it includes banana, strawberry, almond milk, and agave nectar. Notice the mixture of sugar from the fruit is supported by proteins from the vegetable green powder. By the way, if you can't find Crystal Manna flakes, substitute green powder from Carolalt.com or E3Live.

Combine all the ingredients in a blender and whir until smooth. Pour and drink.

39 ALEXEI YASHIN'S FROZEN FRUIT DRINK

Juice of 4 oranges

1 ripe banana

5 fresh strawberries, frozen

5 fresh pineapple chunks, frozen

5 fresh mango chunks, frozen

Handful of fresh raspberries, frozen

2 cups purified water, as needed

TIP

For more nutrients and a slightly different taste, you can substitute fresh young coconut milk for regular water. You can freeze your own seasonal fresh fruit or do what Alexei does: keep bags of frozen organic fruit in the freezer so you can make this drink any time

SERVES 2

Again, notice I mix water into this drink to soften the sugar rush somewhat. If he's taking this drink as a meal, Alexei adds green powder to help him sustain the energy he needs over a long period. If he's taking it when he's about to eat, or after he has eaten, he doesn't need the greens. Fruits shouldn't be eaten right before or after solid food because fruit is digested slowly and ferments in the stomach and may make you feel bloated.

I've made this drink more times than I can count because it's the staple Alexei drinks nearly every day. If it can get a professional hockey player charged up, it'll get you going, too!

Combine all the fruit in the blender and whir to combine, adding enough water to make the drink smooth, but not so much that it becomes too thin.

40 SWEET, SWEET, FRESH-SQUEEZED ORANGE JUICE

3 organic oranges

Purified water, as needed

SERVES 1

Last, but surely not least, and simple as can be, here's the juice you have always wanted but probably never had! Time and time again people have told me that they buy the "not from concentrate" OJ in the supermarket, thinking it's fresh juice. Read the label closely; that juice is pasteurized. That's right, it's cooked orange juice, not fresh. Orange juice is a great American staple that's ideal with your breakfast of hearty cereal. (Just remember to mix with a little water to cut the sugar.)

Cut the oranges in half and squeeze them. Depending on their size, they will make a larger or smaller glass for one. Add water according to taste.

▪▪▪▪▪▪ DONALD GOOD AND FAMILY   AML (LEUKEMIA), ALLERGIES, HYPOTHYROIDISM, AND DEPRESSION

"What, me? *Cancer?*"

Elida, Ohio

Donny Good could hardly believe his ears.

The twenty-five-year-old husband and father hadn't been his usual strong-as-an-ox self lately. It started in November 2005. He lost his appetite and was feeling unusually tired. He began vomiting in the evenings. At first his wife, Nicole, thought that maybe he was simply working too hard and wasn't getting enough sleep. But by December he had lost a lot of weight, going from 190 pounds down to 170. As the days passed he became weaker and weaker. Some days at work, where he drove a dump truck at an excavation site, he found himself falling asleep at the wheel. Taking vitamins didn't help. He didn't know what to do.

"I had been a bodybuilder since I was fifteen. I considered myself pretty healthy," he says. Growing up in a close-knit, traditional Mennonite family in rural Ohio, Donny was unafraid of long hours of manual labor. Yes, he had been working hard, but that clearly wasn't the problem.

By Christmas he could hardly move. He literally had trouble putting one foot in front of the other. Donny needed to see a doctor. On January 12 he did, and that's when the doctor gave the Good family the unimaginable news. Results from a blood test showed that Donny was suffering from acute myelogenous leukemia (AML), a fast-growing cancer of the blood and bone marrow.

"The shock and devastation that hit us was something I never want to experience again. It seemed like time stopped. We could not even grasp what the doctor was saying," Donny recalls.

The doctor recommended that Donny go to Ohio State University Comprehensive Cancer Center, the James Cancer Hospital, in Columbus, Ohio, as soon as possible. He went the very next day and was admitted.

"My leukemia was a very severe type, M5. The doctors said that they needed to treat it aggressively if I was going to have any chance to live. To begin with, they recommended a very strong dose of chemotherapy. They wanted to see if they could get the leukemia under control first; then, they said, they would need to do a bone marrow transplant," Donny recalls.

"We struggled so hard those first few days," Donny says. "I found myself asking God, 'Why? Why us? Why me? God, we are young. We are just starting our life together.'"

Family and friends, especially from their church, rallied around the Goods. His wife's cousin took care of the Goods' home and their pets. If Donny lived, it would be a long haul. As a young family they didn't have a lot of their own resources to fall back on. But people visited at the hospital and brought gifts—more than enough to pay the mortgage. According to Donny, "It seemed like God was saying, 'See, I am still here to take care of you. Trust in me.'"

Donny spent a full month in the hospital. His treatments were grueling, painful, and in their own way made Donny sicker. At times he felt that he would die from the regimen of chemotherapy rather than the disease. He was so weak that he didn't have the strength to hold his four-month-old son, Dallas. He even needed help to turn over in bed. He had lost another twenty pounds. But when he was released on February 14 it was the happiest Valentine's Day of his life. He was not well, but least he was alive!

Before leaving the hospital, however, doctors told Donny that no matter what, he needed a bone marrow transplant if he was to survive. After a short hiatus at home, until a transplant donor could be identified, they wanted him to continue receiving chemotherapy.

Donny returned to the hospital once again in March only to learn that neither his brother nor his two sisters were a match for a transplant. The next option was to go to the National Bone Marrow registry in hopes of finding someone. Meanwhile, the best course of treatment was more chemo.

"The thought occurred to me: What if they don't find a donor? What if there is no match? At first the thought was terrifying to me. Then I began to wonder: What if there is another way to fight this without the use of toxic chemicals? And as I did more research into bone marrow transplants I began to wonder if I wanted to go through with it or not. I called out to God and asked him to show me if there was another way to fight this battle. Looking back, I know God answered my prayer," Donny says.

A series of events led him to consider alternatives to the conventional treatments. "Almost everything I was reading talked about raw food and the benefits of eating and drinking organic raw fruits and vegetables," Donny recalls. "I began to realize how the live enzymes in raw food feed the body and build the immune system, which helps to fight diseases. The chemotherapy I was taking was destroying my immune system instead of building it up. The problem with my body was not the lack of chemotherapy, which is toxic poison, but rather the lack of proper nutrition and live enzymes."

He started by refusing the cooked meals that were being served in the hospital. His wife Nicole brought in raw organic food instead, set up a little kitchen in his room and prepared his meals each day.

After three and a half weeks in the hospital, Donny went home once again, still uncertain if he would go through with a transplant, or even if one would become available. He was scheduled to return to Columbus in a month and wouldn't know anything new before then. Meanwhile, Nicole served Donny only raw organic foods and he started juicing. Before long he was consuming three quarts of fresh vegetable juice, five quarts of distilled water, and three complete raw meals a day. Each day he lay out in the sun for twenty minutes. He started exercising by walking half a mile. He also spent time praying and meditating daily and by 9:30 each evening he was in bed.

On returning to the hospital, the Goods got some important news. There still was no bone marrow match for Donny.

"Instead of the disappointment, fear, and despair I thought I would feel, I was almost glad. I now knew what it was going to take to get my body better. Food would be my medicine," says Donny.

But there was still more news. Results of a bone marrow biopsy showed no sign of leukemia. None. Everyone was amazed. Still, the doctors wanted to do four or five more rounds of chemo immediately. The leukemia could come back at any time, they told him. Without more chemotherapy, Donny's chances of survival were still only 20 percent, they said. But feeling so much better, and convinced that he was making the right decision, he refused the treatments. He returned home hopeful and determined to continue getting better.

Since March 2005, the Good family has continued to eat almost completely raw. Donny now walks two to three miles a day and has gained back the forty pounds he lost. He keeps to his daily schedule. Determined to rebuild his immune system, Donny has not returned to work yet, but he feels strong. "I know it's hard to believe, but I feel better today than I ever have," he says. Besides raw food, he credits the family and church community support he has received, and God, for his getting well.

Donny Good's eating raw has not only helped him beat cancer. It has helped turn around his family's health, too. "My wife used to suffer from such severe allergies that one time four years ago when she was walking through a field she went into ana-phylactic shock, but since she has been eating raw they have entirely vanished. My one-and-a-half-year-old son, Dallas, has never eaten cooked food and, unlike most kids, he has never been sick, never even had a cold," says Donny.

His sister Michele, who lives ten hours away in Pennsylvania, was already im-pressed by what she heard about Donny when she met writer David Roth. He intro-duced her to *Eating in the Raw.* Michele sent copies of the book to Donny and their parents. Michele had her own health problems. Perhaps eating raw food could help her, too, she thought. She was being treated for hypothyroidism and depression. After reading the book she started preparing the recipes in it to feed herself. Very quickly she could feel a change. Her chronic lethargy, one of the telltale signs of un-deractive thyroid, disappeared; she felt a new energy. Her overall mood was chang-ing for the better, too. After one month of eating raw she was able to discontinue her antidepressant and by August was off her thyroid medication.

Growing up, the Good family ate like everyone else around them. Coming from a rural farming community, the quality of their food was probably better than most Americans'—but it was cooked. Today, in their sixties, Donny and Michele's parents have begun to change the way they're eating too. There are more raw foods in their diet. Though it may seem hard to change old ways, sometimes it's worth it and for the better.

"After all we have been through and all we have experienced, my family and I will never go back to the standard American diet," Donny says.

10 RAW SNACKS

In *Eating in the Raw* I described how my family ate when I was a child. One of the things I remember vividly was the important role snack food played in our day-to-day lives. Some of the snacks were sweet, and some were salty, and of course, most of them were bad for us. **Snack food was what you ate when you hung around with friends and relaxed; it was a big part of socializing.** Even now, when you visit the Alts there are always plenty of things to nosh on. We Alts really love our snacks!

So I wasn't surprised when, shortly after my sister Christine started to eat raw, she turned her attention to developing raw replacements for the snacks we grew up with. The big difference is that now we can enjoy them without guilt. And they're just as delicious as ever!

The best part is that these snacks are good for you. As I mentioned before, when you deal with raw foods, you have to discard everything you know about food because raw is not the same as cooked, and it has a different effect on the body. I love to tell people that my granola has more nutritious fruits and nuts and spices in it and is better for them than a plate of pasta! Can you imagine telling your kids, don't eat dinner, eat your trail mix? Go on and make a big batch of granola and let the kids go wild on it. Let them ruin their appetites for once. At least they're ruining it with healthy food!

As an aside: While eating a bowl of One Lucky Duck's amazing raw ice cream the other night, I watched VH-1's *100 Best Bodies*. I saw all these poor celebs working out day in, day out. It seemed so ironic that they struggle with their physiques just so they can eat unhealthy cooked foods, while I eat healthy, guilt-free ice cream in the comfort of my chair! That is the raw-food difference in a nutshell.

If you find you don't have the time to make snacks yourself, then try an online source. Good Stuff by Mom and Me and Raw Revolution are just two of the companies making great healthy snacks.

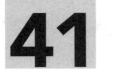

41 CHEESE, CRACKER, AND PEAR PLATE

FLAX CRAX

1 pound flax seeds, soaked for 3 to 4 hours

1 cup Bragg Liquid Aminos or Nama Shoyu

2½ cups purified water

Raw cheddar, brick, bouche, and smethe (Camembert-like) cheeses

Fresh, ripe organic pears

This seems like a no-brainer: cheese and crackers. But many people don't realize that just because a food is sold cold, it doesn't mean it's not cooked. Cheese is the perfect example. The milk in cheese is usually cooked or pasteurized. So the cheese itself is cold, but the ingredients are cooked. But once again, if you read the labels, you will find that some cheeses are labeled "raw-milk" cheeses. These are the cheeses you should look for. So ask your cheese expert what is what and they will tell you.

Grind the flax seeds in a spice grinder, coffee grinder, or blender, and transfer to a bowl. Add the Bragg Liquid Aminos or Nama Shoyu and let stand for at least 30 minutes. The batter should be thick and spreadable. If necessary, add some of the water.

Spread the batter on Teflex-lined dehydrator trays about an ⅛ inch thick and dehydrate for 8 hours or overnight. Then flip the crackers over, peel off the Teflex sheets, and return to the dehydrator until completely dry and crispy, about 2 to 3 hours more. Store leftover crackers in an airtight container.

Cut the cheeses into wedges and arrange on a platter. Core and quarter the pears and arrange around the cheese. Add the crackers and serve.

42 CHRISTINE'S IT'S-CHEESE CRACKERS

3 cups fresh corn kernels, or frozen corn, thawed

2 cups shredded raw organic cheddar cheese, mild or sharp, loosely packed

1 red, orange, or yellow bell pepper, seeded and chopped

2 tablespoons chopped red onion

¼ teaspoon cayenne pepper

¼ teaspoon chili powder

¼ teaspoon Himalayan salt

The ever popular Cheez-It was a favorite in our house. So naturally my sister and I found a raw alternative. This only proves what I tell people when they ask me how I can stay on a raw lifestyle—whatever you eat cooked, I can find it for you raw.

Combine all the ingredients in a food processor or blender and process until the corn is pulverized and the mixture is well blended. Spread onto Teflex-lined dehydrator trays and place in the dehydrator. Dehydrate at 115 degrees F for approximately 6 hours or until the tops are dry to the touch. Flip over the crackers onto the dehydrator trays, and peel off the Teflex liners. Dehydrate for approximately 6 more hours, or until the tops are a bit drier.

Cut into small cracker-size squares and return to the dehydrator, approximately 10 to 20 hours longer, depending on how crunchy you would like them. I prefer this cracker on the chewy side, not on the crispy side, so I dehydrate for less time, approximately 20 hours total.

43 MURIEL'S STICKY GRANOLA

3 cups mixed raw nuts and seeds, such as buckwheat, walnuts, sliced almonds, pumpkin seeds, and sunflower seeds, germinated (see pages 41–43)

½ cup raw honey

2 tablespoons ground cinnamon

5 pitted dates

¼ cup raisins

TIPS

If you really like a cinnamon flavor, when the granola is dehydrated, but still sticky, place it in a resealable plastic bag and sprinkle with more cinnamon. Shake to distribute it. This also works well with coconut flakes, for a more tropical mixture.

If you can't find raw sliced almonds and wish to use raw whole almonds, put the whole almonds in the food processor alone and pulse them a few times before adding other ingredients.

MAKES 5 CUPS

I eat this nearly every day, either to snack on or for a meal. Remember, when making this, however, the nuts and seeds all germinate at different times. So make sure you note the time you must dump off the water and put a certain nut or seed into the refrigerator while waiting for the longer-germinating nuts or seeds to finish. The cold of the refrigerator slows down the enzyme action in the seeds, allowing you to keep them fresh until all your seeds or nuts are done.

Put the mixed nuts and seeds in the food processor and pulse a few times to pulverize. Mix the honey and cinnamon in a large bowl. Add the nut and seed mixture and toss to combine. Chop the dates into small pieces and add to the nuts, along with the raisins.

Spread the mixture on Teflex-lined dehydrator trays and dehydrate at 115 degrees F for approximately 12 hours, or until the mixture is the desired stickiness.

Variations Here are some other good flavor combos to consider: **Coconut and dried banana slices** • **Coconut and dried pineapple slices** • **Coconut, dried pineapple, dried banana, and ground ginger** • **Hazelnuts and vanilla extract** • **Cacao nibs and almond extract** • **Dried mangos and orange rind**

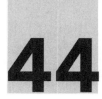

44 AWESOME FOODS' CASHEW CHEESE SPREAD

10 ounces raw cashews

½ cup plus 2 tablespoons purified water

1 yellow bell pepper, seeded and cut into chunks

5 tablespoons fresh lemon juice

½ cup dried parsley

1½ tablespoons chopped fresh dill

1½ teaspoons dried basil

1 teaspoon freshly ground black pepper

1 teaspoon granulated garlic

1 teaspoon granulated onion

¼ teaspoon raw sesame seeds

Scant ¼ teaspoon Himalayan salt

Assorted crackers for serving

MAKES 2 CUPS

Remember when I told you that cashews are versatile? Here is another case in point. We have had cashews in desserts, dinners, and now here they are as a snack. We'll do roasted, salted, and spicy nuts later in this chapter.

This spread, and the tomato variation that follows, both come from Awesome Foods, Bruce Weinstein's raw food company in Bridgeport, Pennsylvania.

Put the cashews in a food processor and process until finely ground. Add the water and process until thick and creamy. Add the remaining ingredients except the crackers and process until smooth. Serve with the crackers of your choice.

Variation: Tomato Cashew Cheese Spread

Soak ⅓ cup of sun-dried tomatoes in water for 4 hours, drain, and finely chop. Add them to the spread along with apple pectin capsules. Mix well and serve as above.

45 SNACK NUT TRIO

CINNA-NUTS

2 teaspoons date powder

¼ cup raw honey

½ teaspoon ground cinnamon

½ teaspoon sea salt

2 cups raw walnuts or other nuts, germinated (see pages 41–43)

MAKES 2½ CUPS

Since my sister Christine is a gourmet cook, I can tell her what I need and she can figure out a raw recipe for it! So these three nut recipes are hers, with a little help from me. Remember, I told you we Alts love snacks. Here she proves my point!

Mix the date powder, honey, cinnamon, and sea salt in large bowl until well combined. Toss in the walnuts and mix until well coated. Spread the nuts on Teflex-lined dehydrator trays and dehydrate at 115 degrees F for 15 to 24 hours until they are sticky but no longer wet. Store the cooled nuts in an airtight container.

TIP

Date powder is just what it seems: powdered dates. If you wish to make your own date powder, just dehydrate the dates (see page 39 for preserves). Then when they are completely dry, break off pieces and grind in a coffee grinder until powdered. Put it in an old salt or sugar shaker for future use.

SPICY MACS

MAKES 2½ CUPS

2 cups raw macadamia nuts

¼ cup raw honey

1 teaspoon cayenne pepper

1 teaspoon sea salt

Germinate the macadamia nuts for 1 hour, rinse, and drain. Mix the honey, cayenne, and sea salt well in large bowl. Toss in the macadamia nuts and coat well with the honey mixture. Spread out the nuts on Teflex-lined dehydrator trays and place in dehydrator at 115 degrees F for 15 to 24 hours until they are sticky but no longer wet. Store the cooled nuts in an airtight container.

SIMPLE SALTED NUTS

MAKES ABOUT 3 CUPS

3 cups raw nuts of your choice germinated (see pages 42–43)

2 teaspoons cold-pressed, extra-virgin olive oil

Himalayan salt to taste

Toss the germinated nuts in the olive oil until well coated and sprinkle with the sea salt. Start off with a little salt at first, and add more to taste. Toss well. Spread out the nuts on Teflex-lined dehydrator trays and dehydrate at 115 degrees F for 6 to 10 hours. If you find the nuts are too oily, dehydrate longer. Place the nuts on a paper towel to soak up any excess oil and salt again. If nuts still seem too oily, use less oil next time.

46 CAROL'S GYM OR TRAIL MIX

1 cup raw sunflower seeds

1 cup raw pumpkin seeds

1 cup raw almonds

1 cup raw macadamia nuts

1 cup broken raw walnuts

1 cup raisins or Goji berries

1 cup raw chocolate (cacao) nibs (optional)

Dash of Himalayan salt (optional)

TIP

See the snack trio on the previous pages if you wish to flavor your trail mix.

MAKES 6 TO 8 CUPS

I want to thank Pam Krauss at Clarkson Potter for this one. I had never thought of doing my own trail mix because I usually order it online. But making it myself gives me the versatility to choose what I put into it. Not only did Pam give me this great idea, she also gave me great suggestions for what to put into it and she named it too. The secret to this mix is to make it the way you like it. I always keep some in my purse.

In separate containers, germinate the sunflower seeds, pumpkin seeds, almonds, and macadamia nuts, but do not germinate the broken walnut pieces. (See the chart on page 43.) Dehydrate the germinated nuts and seeds thoroughly at 115 degrees F until they're crunchy again (at least 24 hours) and cool to room temperature. Mix the dehydrated nuts with the walnut pieces, raisins or Goji berries, and chocolate if using. Sprinkle with salt if desired and store in an airtight container.

47 CHRISTINE'S HUMMUS

1 cup raw dried chickpeas

Juice from ½ lemon

3 tablespoons cold-pressed, extra-virgin olive oil

5 tablespoons purified water

½ cup raw sesame tahini

2 small or 1 large garlic clove, minced

½ teaspoon Himalayan salt

Kelly's Super Flax Crax (page 96) or another flax seed cracker for serving

TIPS

Tahini is sesame paste. In the store read the label because the raw version is probably right next to the cooked one. Look for the word "raw" on the label.

This hummus is best after it sits overnight in the refrigerator.

MAKES 2½ CUPS

Hummus is another example of a cold food that might not actually be raw. The hummus you buy at the deli is in the refrigerated section, but all its main ingredients are cooked: the chickpeas, oil, and, I'm pretty sure, the tahini too, depending on the hummus you choose. Allow me this opportunity to pass along something that Dr. Timothy Brantley told me: the heat used to cook the chickpeas changes their molecular structure, changing the ratio of proteins to carbohydrates. Before it is cooked there are more proteins; after, there are more carbs. This doesn't happen just with chickpeas, but with all legumes. Think about that the next time you order lentil soup. No more protein; you are eating a carbohydrate, of which the body needs very little. And the oils that they use in hummus are cooked too, thereby making them, more or less, rancid trans-fatty acids (i.e., fattening).

Soak the chickpeas for 8 hours, or overnight. Drain the chickpeas and combine in a food processor or blender with the lemon juice, oil, water, tahini, garlic, and salt. Process until the chickpeas are ground up and all the ingredients are well mixed and creamy. If you find the mixture is too thick, slowly add more water while blending. Serve with your favorite flax seed crackers.

48 CAROL'S "CAN'T LIVE WITHOUT IT" TOMATO SOUP

About 8 ounces hot, but not too hot, purified water

2 tablespoons raw tomato concentrate

2 tablespoons Quantum-Rx Nutritional Flakes

1 tablespoon Quantum Medi-Aminos

¼ teaspoon coral calcium

2 dashes Udo's Choice Oil (or Quantum-Rx EFA Oil Blend)

Salt to taste

TIP

When I'm traveling, I buy distilled bottled water. I try to get it in glass bottles because the cloudy plastic ones leach chemicals into the water.

SERVES 1

When I'm traveling I can't always get a good, home-uncooked meal when I want it, but after all these years of eating raw, I've learned how to take care of myself. I always keep a supply of raw snacks with me, but my real ace in the hole is this ultra-nutritious tomato soup. I mix these ingredients in one jar or plastic bag and carry it with me when I'm on the road so that wherever I am, any time of day or night, I can have a quick cup of the soup I simply can't live without. Just add warm water!

In a small pan, heat the water until warm, no more than 115 degrees F. Add the tomato concentrate and the remaining ingredients and stir to combine.

49 CHIPS 'N' DIPS

RAW CORN CHIPS

6 ears corn

½ onion, quartered

2 cups sunflower seeds

1½ tablespoons Bragg Liquid Aminos

½ teaspoon Himalayan salt

¼ cup purified water

MAKES 8 CUPS LOOSELY PACKED CHIPS

What will they think of to make raw next? I hope popcorn, because at this point that's really my only cooked weakness with no raw cousin! You can order raw corn chips online, but they're expensive. These corn chips are easy to make, so best to whip 'em up yourself. The mixing takes but a second. The dehydrating, as usual, takes longer.

Cut the kernels from the corn cobs and put the fresh corn in a blender or a food processor with the onion. Process them until smooth, and then add the sunflower seeds, Bragg Liquid Aminos, and salt. Continue to blend until smooth. If the batter is too thick and clumpy, add a little purified water.

To make the chips, use a teaspoon to scoop the batter onto a Teflex-lined dehydrator tray, flattening each mound to make it about ⅛ inch thick and 1½ inches wide. Dehydrate at 105 degrees F for 12 hours, then remove the Teflex sheet and turn the chips over onto the tray. Dehydrate for another 10 to 12 hours, or until the chips reach the desired crispness. Cool before serving or storing them in an airtight container.

MANGO **SALSA**

MAKES 2 CUPS
You may serve this salsa right away, but it's best the next day.

3 large ripe mangos, peeled

½ jalapeño pepper with seeds, finely minced

4 scallions, thinly sliced

3 tablespoons chopped fresh cilantro leaves

2 tablespoons lime juice

Cut the mango flesh away from the seed and chop into small, irregular chunks. Put in a medium bowl and stir in the jalapeño, scallions, cilantro, and lime juice until combined. Cover and refrigerate.

ZESTY **GUACAMOLE**

MAKES 3 CUPS

When I buy avocados, I buy them in all stages of ripeness. First I choose very soft ones (squeeze them lightly; if they give under the fingers, they are ripe). Then I look for avocados that are a little harder, and some that are a lot harder. That way, they don't all ripen at the same time, and I don't keep going to the store.

Remember to put your avocados into a brown paper bag and into a dark cupboard to ripen them. But don't forget they're there, which I've done more than once, and boy, what a mess. Now, I put a little "stick 'em" note on the cupboard door to remind myself to check on the avocados.

3 ripe Hass avocados, pitted

1 red onion, diced

3 ripe plum tomatoes, diced

2 fresh cilantro sprigs, stemmed and finely chopped

Juice of 1 lime

Cayenne pepper to taste

Himalayan salt to taste

TIP
Refrigerate the ingredients before making the guacamole if you like yours cool and refreshing.

Scoop the meat from the avocado skins and cut it into chunks. Stir in the onion, tomatoes, and cilantro. Mash the mixture until semismooth, then add the lime juice, cayenne pepper, and salt. Serve right away.

50 ONE LUCKY DUCK'S RAW ICE CREAM

2 cups raw cashews, soaked for approximately 2 hours and drained

2 cups fresh coconut meat or milk

1 cup coconut juice

½ cup raw honey or raw agave nectar

½ cup raw virgin coconut butter/oil

2 tablespoons vanilla extract

Seeds of ½ vanilla bean, or 2 more teaspoons vanilla extract

½ teaspoon salt, or to taste

TIP

I always keep several pints of One Lucky Duck ice cream in my freezer so I never run out. There is always somebody I want to astonish with an ice cream that tastes better than the sum of its nondairy parts. To tell you the truth, I wonder how I ever lived without it.

MAKES 8 CUPS

Sarma Melngailis of One Lucky Duck is rightly famous and not just for her raw ice cream—she is also a raw beauty! This ice cream is amazing, and everyone I take to Pure Food and Wine Restaurant agrees that Sarma's is the best raw ice cream in the world. This recipe is one of several that she makes. It first appeared in the book she co-authored, Raw Food Real World *(2005). Make it! You're in for a surprise and a real treat, whether you serve it as a dessert or you eat it as the most sumptuous of snacks. It's delicious and healthy.*

Put all the ingredients in a blender and puree until very smooth. Pour the mixture into an ice cream freezer and freeze according to the manufacturer's directions. Serve right away or store in the freezer while still firm.

Variations This recipe can serve as the base for other flavored ice creams. Here are a couple of my favorites:

For Chocolate Cinnamon Ice Cream, add 3 tablespoons of raw cacao powder and 1 tablespoon of ground cinnamon before blending.

For Blue Blueberry Ice Cream, omit the vanilla bean and extract, and add ½ cup fresh blueberries before blending.

GLEN MOSES

OVERWEIGHT AND HIGH BLOOD PRESSURE
The Woodlands, Texas

For Glen Moses the turning point came five years ago, at his sister's wedding.

"I was talking with guests at the reception, when I overheard a raw foodist telling unbelievable stories about the benefits of eating raw and how people's lives had been dramatically changed. I had never heard anything like it," Glen recalls.

"At that point in my life I was overweight and had high blood pressure. I really didn't know what to do about it," he admits. A little overwhelmed by what he was hearing, he shared his situation with his new acquaintance, and what he heard gave him hope: "Glen, you can get rid of your high blood pressure if you only eat a 100 percent raw vegan diet."

Glen was intrigued but remained skeptical. He went to see his doctor, who simply wrote him a prescription for blood pressure medication. But Glen couldn't get the raw foodist's challenge out of his mind. Rather than filling the prescription, he decided to try eating entirely raw just for a trial period. His blood pressure rapidly started to go down. Soon it was normal. His weight dropped quickly too.

"I weighed 218 pounds when I started eating raw. My waist was thirty-eight inches. In eight months, without trying to lose weight and without starving myself, I lost eight inches in my waist and weighed 150," says Glen, who is five foot ten.

Although very slim, Glen knew that he was still considered in the healthy-normal range for someone of his height and build, and he felt great. But sometimes his energy level was a little low and some friends and family members were concerned about him. They had never seen Glen so thin.

"On Thanksgiving Day, after months of my loved ones telling me I was too skinny, I decided to join everyone and eat the holiday meal that my aunt had prepared. That was the end of my 100 percent raw diet. From the minute I sat down to that turkey and dressing, I found myself eating cooked food more and more, going from totally raw to about 50 percent raw pretty much overnight," Glen says. Within a short time his weight started rising again and with it, his blood pressure. Memories of his former fat and unhealthy state were all he needed to return to eating raw—this time for good.

"My blood pressure is normal again and I don't take any medications," says Glen. "I'm not as thin as I was when I first went raw, and my weight has settled at about

185. I now eat between 90 and 99 percent raw, though I'm no longer vegan. I always loved chocolate, so of course I love raw cacao nibs now, and also raw honey. The fact is that I don't worry about what I eat these days—so long as it's raw. I feel healthy. Life is good.

AMANDA SAGER

Even as a kid, Amanda Sager was curious about food. Now in her mid-twenties, she's a registered dietitian—and a raw foodist.

DEPRESSION, OVERWEIGHT, AND LOW ENERGY LEVEL

Rochester, New York

Amanda's moment of truth came when she was in college and just happened to be listening to the radio.

"Who knew that Howard Stern would change my life?" she asks. "I turned on the radio and Howard was interviewing some guy who ate only raw foods. It was David Wolfe, not a name I had ever heard before. At first it seemed like the strangest thing I had ever heard of, but as I listened, something within me said 'that makes total sense.' I had to find out more."

Doing homework on food was nothing new for Amanda. Ever since she was a girl she had been reading books about diet and nutrition. "Everyone in my family is heavy, and I decided when I was very young that I didn't want to be, so I would go to the library and get books about food and I read anything I could. I just keep reading and reading," she says.

In college, Amanda exercised regularly and ate what is commonly considered "a balanced diet." She had been a vegetarian since age sixteen and became completely vegan at twenty, but Amanda knew she was still not right with food. "I always had this feeling that my diet was not working. I was overweight, puffy, and pale. My emotions were all over the place, and I was often depressed without good reason or explanation. My energy level was low, and I felt somewhat trapped by my eating habits. It's frustrating to think you are following the healthiest diet and then realize you are not," she says. Fascinated, but not entirely convinced that raw food was the answer, she logged on to the Internet and started reading. She went to David Wolfe's website. She contacted raw foodists.

At first Amanda thought those who ate raw food were idealistic phonies, out of touch with the world. Giving up cooked food seemed drastic and ridiculous. But as she read more and heard more stories of people whose lives had been changed by eating raw, she found herself reconsidering.

"At first I was kind of angry that it made such sense to eat raw," she recalls. Now she sees it as a precious truth, hidden but obvious.

The truth that Amanda discovered has to do with how our bodies metabolize food. "It reminds me of when Dorothy from *The Wizard of Oz* was told, 'You had what you needed all along,' because it's not the food that heals us, it is our bodies. Raw food lets us function right—sometimes for the first time," says Amanda.

While at school, Amanda started experimenting with eating more and more raw food. "It's hard in college," she says, "but by the time I was a senior, I was getting close to being totally raw." The encouragement she needed to continue came from the positive changes she saw in herself: weight loss, healthier hair, clear skin, stable moods, and a positive outlook on life. For the first time in her life, she experienced a deep, new sense of freedom that is still with her. "I don't feel addicted to food as I did growing up. Raw food doesn't make you feel that pull," she says.

With a degree in nutrition in hand, Amanda became a registered dietitian and accepted a commission as an officer in the US Air Force. Today, Captain Sager is the service's point-of-contact for vegetarian, vegan, and raw food diets. She advises those who are interested in these diets in compliance with science-based guidelines of the American Dietetic Association. The Air Force doesn't promote them in particular but, through Amanda, offers and supports them. Amanda takes pride in working with a large, diverse group of people to help them include more nutrient-rich plant foods and improve their diets. For Amanda, helping others to make changes in their diet is definitely worthwhile, but it still leaves her hungry to do more. She longs to study and do original research into the effects of raw foods on the human body. "There is so much we just don't know about raw-food nutrition simply because there is not a large volume of research available," she says. Fully understood or not, the lasting, tangible benefits of eating raw are something Amanda sees and feels in her own life every day. "That's why I'm never turning back," she says.

RECIPE CREDITS

Thanks to my sister, Christine, and my mother, Muriel, for allowing me to share so many of their amazing raw recipes. Thanks also to the following people for contributing recipes to *The Raw 50*:

MICHAEL CRESSOTTI OF SUSHI SAMBA: Chilled Watermelon Soup; Sashimi Ceviche; Shaved Asparagus Salad

MELISSA DAVISON: Veggie Kebabs with Barbecue Sauce; Jica-Rice Fresh; Avo-Corn Stuffed Tomato; Mango de Flan; Autumn Chi-lee

CHRISTOPHER DOBROWOLSKI: live live Almond Nut Milk; Yummy Choco-coco Mousse

CASSANDRA DURHAM: Lemon Ginger Coconut Tart

CHARLENE EDGERTON: Creamy Black Pepper and Sage Dressing

MARGI ENDE: Simple Favorite Green Smoothie; Spinach Strawberry Salad with Raspberry Dressing

RAW CHEF DAN HOYT: Cashew Banana Shake; Sprouted Kamut Buns or Flatbread; Arugula Veggie Soup; Cucumber Avocado Soup; "Easy As Pie" Cool Lemon Pie; "Sautéed" Veggies; Coconut Crusted "Shrimp" with Red Curry Sauce; Almond Coconut Cookies; Broccoli Cheddar Cannelloni; Spiced Squash; Quintessence Vanilla Pudding with Fresh Berries; Quintessence Vanilla Avocado Milk; Sweet Cucumber Summer Juice

JANICE INNELLA: Asian Anise Soup; Red Pepper Curry Soup; Tuscan Bread

DAVID JUBB: Ginger Warmer

JACK LALANNE: Energy Boost Drink

BRIAN LUCAS (CHEF BELIVE LIGHT): Stuffed Bell Peppers

MASON MAHAFFEY: Blueberry Banana Smoothie

SARMA MELNGAILIS: Red Beet Ravioli Stuffed with Tarragon "Goat Cheese"; Baby Spinach and Arugula Salad with Cinnamon Balsamic Dressing and Candied Walnuts; Strawberry Tart; One Lucky Duck Raw Ice Cream

LISA MONTGOMERY: Three-Nut Pesto Pasta

JOHN MORETTI: Fountain of Youth Sweet Cucumber Summer Juice

VITO NATALE: Fruit and Chocolate Decadence; Frozen Watermelon Cheesecake; Amazing Brownies

TRACEY ODDO: Raw Egg Mayonnaise

HEATHER PACE: Raw Lasagna; Banana Berry Tart

KELLYANN PALAZZOLO: Baby Spinach Salad with Carrot Horseradish Dressing; Beet and Apple Salad

MARTIN ROTH: Favorite Cole Slaw

KELLY SERBONICH: Meatless Meatloaf; Red Pepper Catsup; Cabbage and Peas Tarragon; Macadamia Whipped Cream; Ideal Meal Salad for One; Super Flax Crax

PENNI SHELTON: Perfect Green Goddess; The Not-So-Green Drink

BRUCE WEINSTEIN: Cashew Cheese Spread/Tomato Cashew Cheese Spread; Spinach Quiche

ALEXEI YASHIN: Frozen Fruit Drink

ACKNOWLEDGMENTS

When you are writing a book, you really find out who your friends are. So, thank you to my friends and my family for helping with this immense project! Thanks to:

Nicholas Gonzalez, M.D., for once again sharing his and his patients' insights, wisdom, knowledge, and experience, and for writing the foreword.

Those who contributed recipes: Especially my sister Christine Alt, who worked overtime with me to make sure I had all the recipes I needed; Christopher Do-browolski of live live & organic New York City, who filled in the gaps; Raw Chef Dan Hoyt of Quintessence Restaurant in New York City, for timely responses and last-minute recipes; Melissa Davison of Terra Bella Cafe in Redondo Beach, for sharing your award-winning creations; Michael Cressotti and the chefs of Sushi Samba; the suburban Philadelphia monthly raw potluckers: Janice Innella—The Beauty Chef, Lisa Montgomery, Vito Natale, and Bruce Weinstein of Awesome Foods; and Cassandra Durham, Charlene Edgerton, Margi Ende, David Jubb of Jubb's Longevity in New York City, Jack LaLanne, Brian Lucas (aka Chef BeLive Light), Mason Mahaffey, Sarma Melngailis of Pure Food and Wine in New York City and oneluckyduck.com, Tracey Oddo, Heather Pace, KellyAnn Palazzolo, Martin Roth, Kelly Serbonich, Penni Shelton, Alexei Yashin, Tatiana Yashin, and my mom, Muriel Alt, who supplied recipes, "lent an ear," and has given me support in this and in everything I have done in my life.

Those who are profiled in *The Raw 50*, and the many other people who shared their knowledge, life stories, and experience of eating raw: Bella AgamaOm, Christine Alt, Jake Andra, Marcelle Angelo, Colette Bizal, Peter Clement, Melissa Davison, Justin Donne, Victoria Ellison, Margi Ende, Rebekah Fraser, Donald Good, Michele Good, Aavigalle Haas, James C. Harwood, Lainey Heller, Kristin Hickey, Jim Igo, Rindi Klarberg, Nora Lenz, Tom Lindsley, Katherine Marion, Nadya Markin, Rachel Maynard, Aldie Mincey, Nicole Misiorowski, Lisa Montgomery, Glen Moses, Susanna Norlund, KellyAnn Palazzolo, Anakalia Robles, Suzanne Roth,

Amanda Sager, Kelly Serbonich, Penni Shelton, Christopher Snow, Karl Starkweather, Ginger Tansen, Marielle Tavares, Yahneen Toombs, Julie Weiss, Kelly Williamson.

Raw food experts who shared information and provided support: Gabriel Cousens, M.D., of the Tree of Life Rejuvenation Center in Patagonia, Arizona, and again my friend Christopher Dobrowolski of live live & organic in New York City, and David Jubb, Ph.D., of Jubb's Longevity in New York City.

Those who worked on the cover photo shoot: photographer Ben Fink, Marysarah Quinn, and Nikki Van Noy; designer Laura Palese; stylist Peter Clement; hair/makeup artist Bata; assistants Margarida Correia, Jeff Kavanaugh, and Joelle Jensen; Beck Preston of Queenie Jewelry (queeniejewelry.com); and Sarma Melngailis and the staff of Pure Food and Wine. A special thanks to Christiano Mancini of Roberto Cavalli in the New York City showroom and press office for the fabulous cover dress!

For food photos: Ryu Kodama of ryukodama.com for his generosity, as well as Melissa Davison, Lisa Montgomery, and Kelly Serbonich. For special assistance: Joanna Cisowska, public relations for Sushi Samba, for getting me recipes, permissions and photos; and, Lynda Gentile of Tristar Products for Jack LaLanne and the Jack LaLanne Power Juicer.

And the people at Clarkson Potter/Random House: My super editor Pam Krauss—thank you for your long nights and personal time spent on this manuscript; Aliza Fogelson, for your patience and troubleshooting; and Kathleen Fleury for accepting countless e-mails.

Penny Simon and Melanie A. Bonvicino for the terrific PR—thanks for touting *both* of my books to the ends of the earth!

Scott Hart, my manager, for always supporting me in all I do.

My patient, supportive, and ingenious agent and friend, Laura Dail of the Laura Dail Literary Agency.

My writer, my friend, and my confidant David Roth—without you there would be no book.

To all: thank you, thank you, thank you!

INDEX